FORENSIC PSYCHOLOGY

RESEARCH,
CLINICAL PRACTICE,
AND APPLICATIONS

MATTHEW T. HUSS

CREIGHTON UNIVERSITY

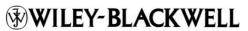

⊛WILEY-BLACKWELL

A John Wiley & Sons, Ltd., Publication

This edition first published 2009
© 2009 Matthew T. Huss

Blackwell Publishing was acquired by John Wiley & Sons in February 2007. Blackwell's publishing program has been merged with Wiley's global Scientific, Technical, and Medical business to form Wiley-Blackwell.

Registered Office
John Wiley & Sons Ltd, The Atrium, Southern Gate, Chichester, West Sussex, PO19 8SQ, United Kingdom

Editorial Offices
350 Main Street, Malden, MA 02148-5020, USA
9600 Garsington Road, Oxford, OX4 2DQ, UK
The Atrium, Southern Gate, Chichester, West Sussex, PO19 8SQ, UK

For details of our global editorial offices, for customer services, and for information about how to apply for permission to reuse the copyright material in this book please see our website at www.wiley.com/wiley-blackwell.

The right of Matthew T. Huss to be identified as the author of this work has been asserted in accordance with the Copyright, Designs and Patents Act 1988.

Wiley also publishes its books in a variety of electronic formats. Some content that appears in print may not be available in electronic books.

Designations used by companies to distinguish their products are often claimed as trademarks. All brand names and product names used in this book are trade names, service marks, trademarks or registered trademarks of their respective owners. The publisher is not associated with any product or vendor mentioned in this book. This publication is designed to provide accurate and authoritative information in regard to the subject matter covered. It is sold on the understanding that the publisher is not engaged in rendering professional services. If professional advice or other expert assistance is required, the services of a competent professional should be sought.

Library of Congress Cataloging-in-Publication Data

Huss, Matthew T.
   Forensic psychology : research, clinical practice, and applications / Matthew T. Huss.
      p. ; cm.
   Includes bibliographical references and index.
      ISBN 978-1-4051-5138-2 (pbk. : alk. paper)   1. Forensic psychology.   I.   Title.
      [DNLM: 1. Forensic Psychiatry–methods.   2. Criminal Psychology–methods.
W 740 H972p 2009]

   RA1148.H87 2009
   614′.15–dc22

                                                                                            2008016046

A catalogue record for this book is available from the British Library.

Set in 11.5 on 13.5 Bembo pt by SNP Best-set Typesetter Ltd., Hong Kong
Printed in Singapore by Fabulous Printers Pte Ltd

1   2009

Brief Contents

FORENSIC PSYCHOLOGY

Contents

Preface

Forensic psychology is becoming increasingly popular both on the graduate and the undergraduate level. However, the very term *forensic psychology* is interpreted differently by scholars and the general public. Some experts in the field use it to describe the broad field of psychology and law that includes the clinical practice of psychology, correctional psychology, police psychology, and non clinical areas of psychology and the law (e.g., jury behavior, eyewitness identification). There are several textbooks available that focus on the broader field. However, there are a lack of quality textbooks that focus solely on the clinical practice of forensic psychology, which is primarily exemplified in the assessment and treatment of individuals who interact with the legal system, for undergraduate students and even beginning graduate students. This textbook is designed to focus on the more narrow or traditional definition of forensic psychology – the practice of forensic clinical psychology. Accordingly, this text has several specific objectives in introducing this field to students.

1. The need for clinical psychologists to practice within their *scope of practice* as a forensic psychologist is emphasized. Scope of practice is defined by adhering to the empirical literature, practicing within one's expertise, and avoiding practice as a legal actor (e.g., attorney, judge, and jury) and instead practicing as a psychologist within the legal context. Throughout the text, scope of practice issues are mentioned and at times explained in great depth. Furthermore, the legal and ethical ramifications for practicing outside one's scope of practice are discussed.
2. Accordingly, the text focuses on empirically supported clinical practice and places little emphasis on aspects of forensic psychology that currently have little empirical support or are purely sensational. It is not within the scope of this text to identify the best clinical practice, but there will be emphasis on the use of research and the need for forensic psychologists to be scholar-practitioners. Part of this emphasis will be to critically evaluate aspects of clinical practice that need greater empirical support.

3. The text also exposes students to case law and statutory law necessary in the practice of forensic psychology. Students should recognize that forensic psychologists need to be familiar with the law in a given jurisdiction in order to be useful to the courts. Significant discussion of case and statutory law also enables students to understand the role of the law in shaping forensic psychology and the lives of people impacted by forensic psychology.

4. This text encourages understanding of the law as a living and breathing entity in the practice of forensic psychology, as in its ability to be therapeutic or anti-therapeutic to the people impacted by it. The term therapeutic jurisprudence is used broadly in this text as a way to anchor students to the importance of the law and is intended to suggest that the law can have negative or positive effects depending on both its original determination and the manner in which it is applied.

5. This text tries to incorporate real world examples that grab the attention of students. Case studies and real world examples are a regular part of the textbook both in terms of special text boxes and integration within the text itself. This objective is especially important in a textbook focusing on the practice of clinical psychology in order to give the student some introductory semblance of the actual practice of forensic psychology.

6. This textbook is intended to be user friendly to students and the instructor. The writing style is intended to be scholarly but engaging to students. Not only is this textbook's focus on the application of forensic psychology but it also focuses on helping students get an accurate understanding of the necessary training/education and available employment opportunities. For the instructor, there are a limited number of primary chapters in order to make the text flexible so that instructors can choose chapters as their own interest/expertise dictates or supplement the text as they desire.

The textbook is organized into five different sections. The first section of the text covers the Fundamentals of Forensic Psychology and includes three chapters. Chapter 1 serves as the primary introductory chapter, What is Forensic Psychology?, and begins to introduce the ideas that students will see throughout the textbook. Chapter 1 focuses on defining what forensic psychology is and what forensic psychology is not. The more sensational aspects of forensic psychology are mentioned along with often inaccurate media depictions. The broader field of psychology and law is referenced but it is made clear that the primary focus of this textbook will be on the clinical practice of forensic psychology. The chapter concludes by discussing the training and education necessary to become a forensic psychologist. Chapter 2, Assessment, Treatment and Consultation in Forensic Psychology, serves as another introductory chapter and describe clinical assessment and treatment broadly and within a forensic context. Specifically, it discusses the unique challenges that

PART I Fundamentals of Forensic Psychology

What is Forensic Psychology? An Introduction

What is Forensic Psychology?

You have opened this book looking forward to learning something about **forensic psychology**, one of the fastest growing areas in all of psychology. But, do you really know what forensic psychology is? Is it like those *Crime Scene Investigation* (CSI) shows on television? Does forensic psychology involve apprehending serial killers? It has to be like the movies! *Silence of the Lambs*? *Kiss the Girls*? These are the types of things forensic psychologists do, right? No doubt theses images portray limited aspects of forensic psychology that tantalize the public. Even though these examples might give inaccurate impressions of forensic psychology, they offer some insight into the field. Ultimately, these images get people interested in the topic and encourage us to think about the horrific things human beings are capable of at their worst.

I rarely tell people when I meet them that I am a forensic psychologist. I usually tell them I work at the local university. My proud father thinks my response makes it sound like I sweep the floors instead of work as a college professor. However, the images that come to mind for the average person when you state that you are a forensic psychologist are sometimes difficult to correct. In this chapter, I am initially going to spend some time clarifying the nature and limits of forensic psychology along with offering a specific definition of forensic psychology that we will use for the remainder of the book. And don't worry; some of those images that come to mind from the movies and television are accurate. Figure 1.1 shows Dr. Theodore Blau, former president of the APA.

Is This Forensic Psychology?

Many people equate forensic psychology with forensic science or law enforcement. They believe that forensic psychologists arrive at a crime scene, survey the area, and eventually identify a number of psychological clues that will help

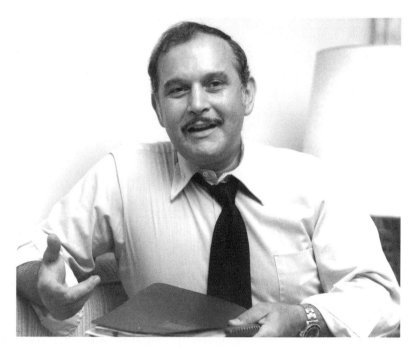

Figure 1.1.   Dr. Theodore Blau, former President of the APA, began working in forensic psychology by testifying as a psychological expert and lectured regularly at the FBI Academy in Quantico, VA. From Psychology Archives – The University of Akron © Skip Gandy, Gandy Photography, Inc., Tampa, FL

catch the criminal. You see these situations continually portrayed by television shows, in the news media, and in movies. In fact, research suggests these media images may be leading to a number of incorrect perceptions about forensic science in general (Patry, Stinson, & Smith, 2008). However, psychologists are not routinely called upon to collect DNA specimens, analyze a sample of dirt left behind for the geographic location from which it originated, or even conduct so called psychological profiles. Forensic psychologists are not biologists or chemists and are rarely crime scene investigators or law enforcement officers. It may sound odd but they are just psychologists. They study human behavior and try to apply those principles to assist the legal system.

When an old friend of mine comes back to town, I often go over to her parents' house for a barbeque. One time her father asked me, knowing that I was a forensic psychologist, "how in the heck do you do therapy with dead people?" Now, while he was at least thinking about forensic psychologists in terms of tasks that psychologists typically perform (i.e., treatment of mental illness), he did not quite have it right when thinking about my work as a forensic psychologist. I don't often channel the dead but it really would be easy to predict the likelihood of future violence for someone who is dead. A number of students come to me interested in using their psychology or criminal justice major and the knowledge of human behavior they have acquired to "catch the bad guys." I usually explain to these students that rarely are forensic psychologists called upon to apprehend suspects; in fact a recent study has found that only about 10% of forensic psychologists and psychiatrists have ever engaged in **criminal profiling** and only about 17% even believe it is a scientifically reliable practice (Torres, Boccaccini, & Miller, 2006). Most students who are interested in catching criminals should look into law enforcement rather than forensic psychology. However, if you are still interested in forensic psychology as a possible career you should know that you do get to spend a considerable amount of time playing detective but more on that later.

The Origin of Forensic Psychology

Part of the public's misconception regarding forensic psychology stems from a lack of awareness about the very origin of the word forensic itself. Although some people think about forensic science and law enforcement when they think of forensic psychology, others might think about high school speech and debate. Focusing on solving arguments or being verbal adversaries in a speech and debate competition actually brings us a little closer to the true meaning of forensic psychology. The word forensic originated from the Latin word *forensis* which means *of the forum* and was used to describe a location in Ancient Rome. The Forum was the location where citizens resolved disputes, something akin to our modern day courtroom, and conducted the business of the day (Blackburn, 1996; Pollock & Webster, 1993). From this context evolved the meaning of forensic psychology. The role of the forensic psychologist is really pretty simple and straight forward, forensic psychologists assist the legal system.

Our Definition of Forensic Psychology

Not only is there confusion in the general public about forensic psychology but there is even debate among psychologists about the nature of forensic psychology (Brigham, 1999). This debate has occurred not only in the United States, where reforms in mental health law and increasing pressure from the courts for clinical testimony have led to growth in the field but also in Canada, Europe, and other parts of the world (Blackburn, 1996; Ogloff, 2004). Broadly speaking, forensic psychology refers to any application of psychology to the legal system. However, many refer to this broader field as *psychology and the law* or *psycholegal studies* while specifying that forensic psychology focuses on the practice of **clinical psychology** to the legal system (e.g., Huss, 2001a). This narrower definition of forensic psychology that focuses only on clinical psychology excludes topics such as eyewitness identification (cognitive psychology), polygraphs (physiological psychology), jury behavior (social psychology), and the testimony of children in court (developmental psychology). These other non-clinical aspects have a powerful impact on the legal system and are extremely important in the psychological study of the law but they are beyond the scope of the current text. Students should check other sources if they have interest in these aspects of psychology and the law (e.g., Brewer & Williams, 2005; Roesch, Hart, & Ogloff, 1999; Schuller & Ogloff, 2001; Weiner & Hess, 2006).

We will focus on a narrower definition of forensic psychology in this book that concentrates solely on the practice of clinical psychology. Our definition of forensic psychology will focus on the intersection of clinical psychology and the law. The clinical practice of psychology generally focuses on the assessment and treatment of individuals within a legal context and includes concepts such as psychopathy, insanity, risk assessment, personal injury, and civil commitment (Huss, 2001b). Furthermore, we will generally avoid topics that are more characteristic of police psychology (criminal profiling, fitness for duty evaluations, hostage negotiation) or correctional psychology that focus on issues pertinent to correctional facilities (prisons and jails) but do not lead to assisting the courts directly.

In using this definition of forensic psychology, we must also differentiate the practice of forensic psychology from forensic psychiatry. Clinical and counseling psychologists are often confused with psychiatrists. Although both psychologists and psychiatrists are trained to assist individuals with mental illness and emotional difficulties in general, there are significant differences (Grisso, 1993). Psychiatrists are medical doctors and obtain MDs or DOs. Psychologists typically obtain PhDs or PsyDs. As a result, psychiatrists are licensed to prescribe medication and emphasize this aspect of patient care. Traditionally, psychologists have not focused on the administration of medication, specifically psychotropic medication, and instead have focused on the psychological assessment and treatment of the mentally ill (see Chapter 2). Psychologists also usually have more extensive training in conducting research (Grisso, 1993) and therefore are better suited to examine many of the ideas we will discuss in this book. There will be issues we focus on that are relevant both to forensic psychology and forensic psychiatry. Nonetheless, we will discuss them from the perspective of the forensic psychologist.

History of Forensic Psychology

Forensic psychology has a deep and extensive history that developed long before popular culture began to focus on it. See Table 1.1 for a brief list of important events in the development of forensic psychology. Hugo Munsterberg is often identified as one of the first psychologists to apply psychological principles to the law in his book, *On the Witness Stand* (1908). The German psychologist, William Stern, also focused on the application of psychological principles to the legal system by studying eyewitness identification in the early 1900s. However, the clinical practice of psychology, as it relates to the legal system, began at about the same time. The clinical practice of forensic psychology originated with Lightner Witmer and William Healy. Witmer began teaching courses on the psychology of crime in the early 1900s and Healy established the Chicago Juvenile Psychopathic Institute in 1909 to treat and assess juvenile

Table 1.1. Important Events in the Development of Forensic Psychology

1908	Publication of *On the Witness Stand* by Hugo Munsterberg
1908	Lightner Witmer teaching courses on the psychology of crime
1909	Establishment of the Chicago Juvenile Psychopathic Institute
1921	Psychologist allowed to testify as an expert witness in *State v. Driver*
1962	Psychologists could testify in cases of insanity in *Jenkins v. United States*
1969	Creation of the American Psychology-Law Society
1970s	Founding of scholarly journals that publish articles exclusive to forensic psychology

delinquents (Blackburn, 1996; Brigham, 1999), thereby serving as the first significant examples of forensic clinical psychologists.

As psychology, specifically the practice of clinical forensic psychology, began to develop in North America during the twentieth century, psychologists were called upon to apply their rudimentary knowledge to the legal system as expert witnesses (see Chapter 3). For example, a psychologist was allowed to testify as an expert witness in the United States in *State v. Driver* (1921) on juvenile delinquency (as cited in Johnstone, Schopp, & Shigaki, 2000). Though the court later rejected the testimony (Johnstone et al., 2000), this event still marked an important step in the development of forensic psychology. Court decisions such as *State v. Driver* tended to legitimize the profession, provided a market for forensic psychologists, and indicated that the legal system sought out psychology as another tool in arriving at fair and just legal outcomes.

However, it was an Appeals Court ruling in the District of Columbia, *Jenkins v. United States* (1962), which marked an even more significant turning point for the entire field of forensic psychology. In *Jenkins*, the court ruled that psychological testimony could be admitted to determine criminal responsibility (i.e., insanity). Forensic psychologists now routinely testify in insanity cases after evaluating defendants. These evaluations are necessary to determine whether defendants exhibit sufficient mental capacity at the time of their crimes to be held responsible for them. Prior to the *Jenkins* ruling, psychological testimony on insanity had largely been excluded in favor of testimony by physicians and psychiatrists (Van Dorsten, 2002). *Jenkins* is one of the first examples in which the law and the legal system influenced both research and the practice of forensic psychology. Specifically, it can be argued that the decision in *Jenkins* led to a boom in forensic psychology in the United States during the 1960s and 1970s because the courts admitted a variety of non-medical testimony (Loh, 1981). Although the Canadian legal system has arguably been less willing to allow psychologists to testify in court, there have been changes in recent years to increase their involvement (Schuller & Ogloff, 2001). Now that psychologists are increasingly being utilized by the legal system, a variety of additional signs point to growth in the field. The largest and possibly most prominent professional organization in forensic psychology, the American Psychology-Law

Society, was first established in 1969 and has grown to over 3,000 members (Grisso, 1991; Otto & Heilbrun, 2002). Furthermore, several forensic related journals in psychology such as *Law and Human Behavior* and *Behavioral Sciences and the Law* began publication in the 1970s (Melton, Huss, & Tomkins, 1999). All of these advances suggest a vibrant and growing profession.

Major Areas of Forensic Psychology

However, the nature of forensic psychology is probably still not totally clear to you. One way to get a better idea about forensic psychology is to examine the major areas of forensic psychology and the law itself. Typically, forensic psychology can be divided into both the criminal aspects and the civil aspects (see Table 1.2 for examples of forensic psychology in both). This division of the roles and tasks of forensic psychology is based on the legal separation between the civil and criminal law. **Criminal law** focuses on acts against society and it is the government that takes the responsibility for pursuing criminal matters through law enforcement officers and prosecutors. The focus of criminal law is to punish offenders in order to maintain a societal sense of justice and deter crime. The murder that may have occurred last night or the mugging down the street are considered violations of criminal law because we, as a society, do not consider these behaviors appropriate and consider violations of criminal law as an offense against any one of us. The state, or the government, acts on behalf of society as the prosecution and files criminal charges against a defendant when it believes an individual has violated the criminal law.

There are a number of legal issues specific to criminal law that often play a role in the practice of forensic psychology. For example, **mens rea** is a principle of criminal responsibility that relates to an individual's mental state. Mens rea, or guilty mind, means that an individual has committed an unlawful act willfully or purposefully. It goes to suggest the culpability or blameworthiness of a defendant. Although psychologists are not called upon to render an opinion in every criminal case as to whether a defendant suffered from a guilty mind, they are called upon in select instances. These instances usually focus on the issue of insanity. In insanity cases, it is the responsibility of the forensic psychologist to assist the court in identifying whether a defendant suffered from a mental

Table 1.2. Example Areas of Forensic Practice in Criminal and Civil Law

Criminal law	Civil law
Risk assessment at the time of sentencing	Child custody
Insanity and criminal responsibility	Civil commitment
Competency to stand trial	Personal injury
Treatment of sexual offenders	Worker's compensation
Juvenile transfer to adult court	Competency to make medical decisions

Key Terms

amicus curiae	criminal profiling	nomothetic
appeals court	district court	policy evaluator
case law	forensic psychology	posttraumatic stress disorder
circuit court	idiographic	stare decisis
civil law	joint-degree program	statutory law
clinical psychology	jurisdiction	therapeutic jurisprudence
common law	mens rea	torts
criminal law		

Further Readings

Bersoff, D. N., Goodman-Delahunty, J., Grisso, J. T., Hans, V. P., Poythress, N. G., & Roesch, R. (1997). Training in law and psychology: Models from the Villanova Conference. *American Psychologist, 52*, 1301–1310.

Packer, I. K., & Borum, R. (2003). Forensic training in practice. In A. M. Goldstein (Ed.), *Handbook of psychology: Vol. 11. Forensic psychology* (pp. 21–32). Hoboken, NJ: Wiley.

2

Assessment, Treatment, and Consultation in Forensic Psychology

So far you have received an introduction to forensic psychology but in this chapter we will take a closer look at the major areas involved in the practice of forensic psychology. Forensic practice can be divided into three specific areas: assessment, treatment, and consultation. The first two areas are not unique to forensic psychology but are central to the practice of clinical psychology and therefore may be somewhat familiar to you if you have had a course in abnormal psychology or clinical psychology. Forensic assessment normally consists of the evaluation of an individual in an attempt to assist the courts in addressing a legal question. As a result there are a number of ethical considerations that are somewhat unique to a forensic assessment (see Chapter 3 for a complete discussion). Forensic assessment relies on similar methods and tools as a general therapeutic assessment but also uses some forensic specific methods. In discussing psychological treatment in a forensic context, we will largely focus on criminal offenders and aspects of treatment that must be especially considered. The third area, consultation, is something that is more likely to occur in forensic practice than routine clinical practice and therefore may be unfamiliar. Consultation is an often ignored but extremely important role for forensic psychologists. Forensic psychologists often assist attorneys or the courts themselves in understanding aspects of human behavior and mental health that do not directly involve the assessment or treatment of individuals. Nevertheless, the consulting forensic psychologist is engaged in a crucial aspect of forensic practice that may be growing in scope and frequency (Andrews, 2005).

Forensic Assessment

When discussing assessment from a clinical psychology perspective (i.e., a therapeutic assessment), the focus is on gathering information about an examinee to make a diagnosis or conclusion about his or her current psychological functioning. This process may mean that when clients walk into a psychologist's office,

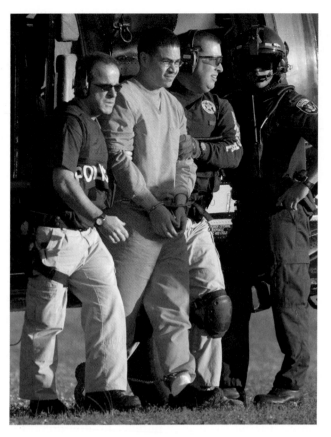

Figure 2.1.   In the case against Jose Padilla, who was accused of plotting a dirty bomb attack in the US, a forensic psychologist assessed Padilla and testified that he suffered from PTSD. © PA Photos / AP.

an emergency room, or a psychiatric hospital that the psychologists interview them, interview other people close to them, examine existing records or administer psychological tests. In forensic assessment, the focus is not only on gathering information that allows the forensic psychologist to make a conclusion about the examinee's mental health but to do so in order to inform the court (Nicholson, 1999). As mentioned previously, these methods are grounded in the same methods that clinical psychologists use to assess anyone presenting with a mental health concern and consist of interviewing, psychological testing, and gathering archival and third party information. The difference is that in a forensic context these methods take on added importance because they have far ranging implications beyond an accurate diagnosis and may extend to the person's freedom or the well-being of society (see Figure 2.1).

Important Tasks in Forensic Assessment

A **therapeutic assessment** is designed to diagnose an individual so that an intervention can be developed and the person's suffering reduced. However, a forensic assessment is different from a traditional therapeutic assessment because there are two additional tasks involved in a forensic assessment. Forensic assessments must clarify and identify the legal question and assess whether forensic psychology has something to offer in a specific situation. Grisso (2003a) has written extensively on the importance of making forensic assessments legally relevant and this will also be a topic we examine at various times.

It is surprising that at times the court or legal parties are not completely clear about their need for a psychologist or the precise legal question to be addressed. An attorney once approached me and stated that his client was as "crazy as a jaybird." It would have been difficult for me to evaluate this examinee to see whether he actually met the threshold requirement for "jaybird craziness." However, after talking more with the attorney it became clear that he was concerned about his client being able to assist him during his trial and his client suffering from a mental illness that would be an important consideration at sentencing, if he was convicted of the crime. There also are times in which the court approaches a forensic psychologist and the forensic psychologist may not have anything to offer the court. For example, there are times in which the psychological literature does not support a legal assumption or strategy. If a prosecuting attorney requests that a forensic psychologist testify that a particular defendant is definitely going to murder someone if he were released, the psychologist would have difficulty doing so because there is not an instrument or assessment approach that can detect, with 100% certainty, that a given individual will commit murder. However, a forensic psychologist would be able to offer an opinion about that individual's overall level of risk, compare him on a risk assessment instrument to other individuals with the same score, and identify the factors that are likely to increase or decrease his risk for future violence. This process is all part of determining what forensic psychology can bring to the assessment process.

Core Concepts in Assessment: Reliability and Validity

Before we discuss specific aspects of therapeutic and forensic assessment, it is important to review two important concepts that are central to assessment and specifically psychological testing. Reliability and validity are terms that can describe the measurement or psychometric soundness of a given test or procedure. **Reliability** generally refers to the consistency of measurement. For example, someone who suffers from depression should obtain a similar score on a psychological test designed to assess depression, like the Beck Depression Inventory-II (BDI-II). If a person is tested from week to week and her symptoms do not change, her scores should be similar each week. If a depressed person's scores vary widely with repeated administrations of the measure while his or her symptoms remain largely unchanged, it would suggest poor reliability for that measure. The scores are not consistent. On the other hand, **validity** is the accuracy of measurement. In order for the BDI-II to be valid it needs to measure depression and not something else. A measure of depression should not measure something like the amount of physical exercise one experiences or something unrelated such as the frequency of watching a television show like *Grey's Anatomy*. Higher levels of both reliability and validity suggest that a procedure or test is sound enough to be used. Reliability and validity are generally expressed by a correlation that ranges from −1 to 1, with a higher correlation indicating better reliability and better validity. One aspect of reliability and validity that is often an issue in forensic assessment is that general clinical procedures and tests are frequently adapted for use in a forensic context without their reliability and validity being properly determined via scientific research (Butcher, 2002). As we will discuss in Chapter 3, this is an issue when we encourage forensic psychologists to practice within their area of expertise or **scope of practice**.

Distinguishing Therapeutic Assessment from Forensic Assessment

Traditional therapeutic or clinical assessments differ from forensic assessments in a number of important ways (Goldstein, 2003). Some of the ways in which they differ include: (1) goals and objectives; (2) relationship of the parties; (3) identity of the client; (4) consequences; and (5) examinee's perspective (see Table 2.1). These differences focus on core overlapping areas between therapeutic and forensic assessments and are in addition to the need for identification of the legal question and assessing whether the forensic psychologist can assist the court.

The first way in which therapeutic assessment differs from forensic assessment is in the *goals and objectives* of each approach. The objective of a therapeutic assessment is to help the examinee by diagnosing and then treating the person for the relevant emotional and psychological problems (Heilbrun, 2003). The objective of a forensic assessment is to assist the court. The forensic psychologist may diagnose an individual with a mental illness but instead of treating that person, the forensic psychologist may simply inform the court how this mental illness impacts the defendant's decision-making or ability to function in a legal

Table 2.1.   Differences Between Therapeutic and Forensic Assessment

	Therapeutic assessment	Forensic assessment
Goals and objectives	Gather information to reduce psychological suffering	Address a legal question
Relationship of parties	One of care and support	Investigative and truth seeking
Identity of client	Client is the examinee	Individual who seeks out and pays for the services
Consequences	Design an intervention	Financial or loss of liberty
Examinee's perspective	Most important source	Heavily scrutinize examinee

context. This difference does not mean the forensic psychologist is without compassion or that the examinee should not or will not be helped, it means that the primary objective in the assessment itself is not to provide information to inform treatment but for some legal purpose.

The *relationship* between the evaluator and the examinee is different in a forensic assessment. In a therapeutic assessment, the role of the therapeutic psychologist is to exhibit concern and offer support. An important part of the therapeutic assessment is to build rapport in order to help the examinee through his emotional difficulties. In a forensic assessment the psychologist adopts more of an investigative role in which he or she is focused on an objective examination of the information pertinent to this examinee (Craig, 2004). Supporting an individual through the legal process or the relevant psychological difficulties is not typically a consideration in the forensic assessment.

It can even be a challenge to determine the *client* in a forensic assessment, a challenge that is not normally present in a therapeutic assessment (Ogloff & Finkelman, 1999). In a therapeutic assessment, the client is very clearly the person who has sought your services. It is the person whom you are evaluating, the person you are interviewing, the person responding to the psychological tests. However, the issue can be more complicated in a forensic assessment. The client or clients may not necessarily be the person sitting across from you in the evaluation because the person who has hired you and to whom you owe a duty is different from the person you are evaluating. In a forensic assessment, the client is more likely to be the court or the attorney who hired you. This difference in the identity of the client is often reflected in the level of confidentiality associated with forensic assessments and the obligation the forensic psychologist has in going further to make the limitations clear while making sure the examinee is giving his or her informed consent for the assessment.

Therapeutic and forensic assessments also differ in the *consequences* of the evaluation (Craig, 2004). The consequences of a therapeutic assessment usually result in an intervention or treatment approach being designed for the examinee. The consequences of a forensic assessment could be a financial reward, a loss of freedom, or even a loss of life. Although the consequences of receiving poor or ineffective treatment should not be minimized, the consequences of a forensic assessment can be more severe.

The accuracy of the information you obtain is generally more questionable in a forensic assessment than in a therapeutic assessment (Melton, Petrila, Poythress, & Slobogin, 1997). During a therapeutic assessment the *examinee's perspective* is heavily relied upon because it is voluntary and there is a shared course of action between the evaluator and the examinee. During a forensic assessment the examinee does not usually present himself voluntarily, the evaluator questions or waits for verification of his statements, and the examinee has something to gain from the outcome of the assessment. As a result, accuracy of the information is much more likely to be at question in a forensic assessment than a therapeutic assessment and the importance of the examinee's perspective varies.

Methods and Procedures: Interviewing

Despite the differences in some of the procedures used in forensic assessment, there also are a number of similarities including the cornerstone of assessment, the clinical interview. Interviewing is the most frequently used method of assessment in psychology and consists of gathering information about an examinee by speaking directly to the examinee. A clinical interview is typically the initial approach used in attempting to gather information about a person because of the ease and depth of information that can be gathered. An interview might last anywhere from a half hour to several hours. Clinical interviews normally consist of asking for personal information about different areas of the examinee's life such as family, work, mental health, substance use, education, or legal involvement. A forensic psychologist might ask a person if he had any difficulties in school with academics, peers, or disciplinary problems. She also might ask the person about his current feelings and thoughts. Is he having any difficulty performing routine tasks such as going to work, hanging out with friends and family, or performing household chores? No matter what specific questions are asked, there are three types of clinical interviews that fall on a continuum from unstructured to structured. In each case, there are certain advantages and disadvantages to using a single approach.

Unstructured interviews

In an **unstructured interview**, the forensic psychologist does not have a prescribed list of questions to ask but instead may have a general idea of the purpose of the evaluation or the areas to focus upon and seek to gather preliminary information. The forensic psychologist may simply ask about the reason for the evaluation and obtain background information that provides a context or explanation. An unstructured interview probably looks very similar whether it is as part of a therapeutic assessment or a forensic assessment.

Unstructured interviews are good for establishing rapport and gathering in-depth information but because of the individual differences between psychologists they may be more inconsistent and less reliable. Establishing rapport means that the psychologist and the examinee are able to get to know one another and that the psychologist is able to construct a situation in which the examinee will be open and honest. We will discuss later why this practice is especially important in forensic assessments and also especially difficult. Nonetheless, it is important to establish rapport so that the examinee gives accurate information freely, whether it is a therapeutic assessment or a forensic assessment. Unstructured interviews also allow the interviewer to follow-up on any response and ask as many additional questions as the interviewer sees as appropriate. However, unstructured interviews tend to be less reliable or consistent in the information they elicit. The questions I ask of a given examinee might be very different from the ones another psychologist asks without a common script. Furthermore, the examinee may give different answers depending on the type of rapport established by each psychologist and the mood of the examinee. There

to testify in the case. In these cases the forensic consultant should become familiar with all aspects of the case in order to be able to give the most comprehensive and useful advice. An attorney may ask a forensic psychologist for information on where to find a psychologist that can testify about the impact of sexual abuse on a child. Moreover, an attorney may not even be aware that a psychological expert could be useful in a given situation or the type of mental health expert that would be the most useful in a particular situation (Drogin & Barrett, 2007). Sometimes consultation consists of educating an attorney on the research in a given area (Gottlieb, 2000). The consultant may be aware of the different accrediting organizations as well as be able to review more competently the past work of potential experts to recommend the best one. An attorney does not have the time to develop this level of knowledge and thereby the forensic consultant can be very useful.

Another common avenue for consultants is to evaluate the testimony or work product of an opposing expert (Singer & Nievod, 1987). A forensic psychologist may review an opposing expert's report to evaluate whether it appears the expert has administered the psychological tests properly, whether the data support the conclusions of the report, and whether the report addresses all of the statutory requirements for the particular civil or criminal issue. An attorney may use this information to cross-examine an opposing expert and identify any errors or questionable issues in a report (Drogin & Barrett, 2007). This task may also involve review of any documentation produced by the expert for the case and anything else the expert has written or stated publicly on the issue. These searches may provide contradictory statements in relevant cases that can be used to discredit the testifying expert.

A final area where forensic psychologists are increasingly being used as consultants relates to policy issues. Many government or independent agencies are using forensic psychologists to help them form policy initiatives or evaluate already existing policy. For example, Norris (2003) explained the role forensic consultants played in reshaping the Catholic Church's policies for the protection of children after the sexual abuse crisis. The Catholic Church formed a commission that was charged with arriving at a set of policies that would protect children from future sexual abuse. Forensic consultants were involved in formulating the new policies and programs and the training of Church officials to implement and respond according to the policies. This example is just one in which forensic consultants can use their expertise outside of the more traditional roles of assessment and treatment.

In addition to these three roles, forensic psychologists are used to consult in numerous other ways outside of testifying as expert witnesses themselves. It should be reiterated that serving as a forensic consultant is a role outside of the normal training that forensic psychologists routinely receive and one that involves potential ethical issues that may conflict with the traditional objective scientific approach taken when serving as an expert. Nonetheless, it is likely that forensic psychologists will increasingly serve as consultants in these traditional roles as well as a host of yet unrecognized roles.

Summary

Forensic assessment tends to be the cornerstone of forensic practice and the most common activity that forensic psychologists perform. Forensic assessments are conducted to assist the court in answering a particular legal question. As a result, forensic assessments tend to differ from traditional therapeutic assessments in several ways: (1) goals and objectives; (2) relationship of the parties; (3) identity of the examinee; (4) consequences; and (5) accuracy of information. Forensic assessments normally consist of a clinical interview that can be unstructured, semi-structured, or structured; psychological testing that may include a variety of psychological tests to assess personality, intelligence, neuropsychological deficits, or even specialized forensic instruments; and a significant reliance on archival and third party information.

Forensic treatment is concerned with treating and rehabilitating a variety of different types of offenders anywhere from violent offenders to mentally disordered offenders. Psychological treatment in forensic settings routinely consists of management, maintenance, outpatient therapy, or programs designed for specific issues relevant to offenders. Treatment of offenders has been controversial both because of the conflicting purposes of the criminal justice system and the mental health system and the mixed evidence for the success of these treatment approaches. Presently, the psychological literature is relatively clear that treatment can be successful and that there are specific components characteristic of successful treatment programs.

The final area of forensic practice is forensic consultation. Forensic consultation includes a variety of informal tasks that can be both distinct from assessment and treatment as well as overlap with them. Because the role of the forensic consultant tends to encourage the forensic psychologist to work as an advocate, certain professional and ethical issues can arise that should be thoughtfully considered.

Key Terms

archival information
cognitive distortions
correctional psychology
criminogenic needs
forensic assessment instruments
forensic relevant instrument
objective tests
projective tests
reliability

responsivity principle
scope of practice
secondary gain
semi-structured interview
specialized forensic instruments
structured interview
therapeutic assessment
unstructured interview
validity

Further Readings

Drogin, E. Y., & Barrett, C. L. (2007). Off the witness stand: The forensic psychologist as consultant. In A. M. Goldstein (Ed.), *Forensic psychology: Emerging topics and expanding roles* (pp. 465–488). Hoboken, NJ: John Wiley & Sons.

Gendreau, P. (1996). Offender rehabilitation: What we know and what needs to be done. *Criminal Justice and Behavior, 23*, 144–161.

Grisso, T. (2003a). *Evaluating competencies: Forensic assessments and instruments*. New York: Kluwer Academic/Plenum Publishers.

3

Expert Testimony and The Role of An Expert

The practice of forensic psychology frequently ends in the forensic psychologist testifying as an expert witness. As an expert witness, psychologists are able to assist the law directly by informing the courts of psychological findings and their application to a particular legal question. However, it is important to remember that forensic psychologists are merely doing just that, assisting the legal system. The legal system and judges in particular are appropriately resistant to their authority being usurped or replaced by psychological evidence (Ogloff & Cronshaw, 2001). The purpose of the forensic psychologist as an expert witness is not to replace the decision-making ability of the court but to assist it. It is also important to realize that forensic psychologists usually serve as experts without testifying in court and much of our discussion in this chapter applies to the testifying expert and the non testifying expert.

By agreeing to enter into the courtroom, psychologists face several important challenges that they otherwise are not exposed to in their routine clinical practice (Brodsky, Caputo, & Domino, 2002). The adversarial nature of the legal system itself is a challenge for forensic psychologists. Psychologists typically practice in environments in which there is collegiality and open discussion of ideas. However, the adversarial nature of the courtroom can make it very clear that ideas and conclusions will not be discussed but instead critiqued in a competitive atmosphere. Furthermore, this criticism is conducted in a very public place and there is little support for the testifying expert. An expert does not have the luxury of calling a timeout or phoning a friend for some helpful advice while on the witness stand. The expert is truly alone. This entire experience takes place in a setting in which the expert is largely unfamiliar and is another reason that expert testimony has been called potentially the most frightening professional experience in psychology (Brodsky et al., 2002).

The increasing use of mental health practitioners as expert witness in the United States, Canada and in many places around the world (Colbach, 1997; Knapp & VandeCreek, 2001; Saunders, 2001) suggests they have a significant impact on the legal system. A. Hess (2006) argues that as our society becomes more complicated and knowledge expands at an exponential rate, there is an even greater need for experts. In fact, he suggests that failure to use an expert in a case could constitute a professional failure on the part of an attorney (Hess, 2006). However, the truth is that the impact of expert testimony on juror decision making is not completely clear (Nietzel, McCarthy, & Kern, 1999). Nietzel and colleagues conducted a **meta-analysis** of 22 published studies examining the impact of expert testimony across a variety of different cases including such diverse topics as child abuse, eyewitness identification, insanity, battered woman or rape trauma syndrome evidence, hypnosis, and polygraph evidence. A meta-analysis is a statistical approach in which the available studies are statistically combined to ask and answer questions that are not possible with only a single study. This statistical approach helps supplement the traditional approach to summarizing an area of research that has consisted of reading the available research and coming to a conclusion based on rational consideration of the different studies. Nietzel et al. (1999) found a modest impact across these different types of cases for expert testimony. Nonetheless, there is no indication that the courts are tired of the testimony of forensic psychologists or will be discontinuing it.

Moreover, the vast majority of forensic work does not culminate in expert testimony. Consultation work by its very nature does not result in testimony as an objective expert. Forensic assessments and treatment also do not tend to conclude in courtroom testimony, probably because the vast majority of cases are settled before trial. Nonetheless, it is still important to focus special attention on testifying experts because much of the public's view of forensic psychology is based on these public displays of forensic work. In addition, many of the issues I will discuss in relation to expert testimony such as ethical concerns and biases are true for any forensic work in which the forensic psychologist is serving as an objective expert, whether it results in courtroom testimony or not.

History of the Expert Witness

Psychologists have not always widely testified as experts. Opinions vary but Gravitz (1995) suggests that one of the first instances of expert testimony in the United States that could be regarded as falling under the general umbrella of forensic psychology or psychiatry occurred in a murder trial in 1846. John Johnson was tried for the murder of Betsey Bolt as part of a plan to cover up a previous sexual assault of Mrs. Bolt by Johnson. An expert, Amariah Brigman, testified extensively on the mental health status of one of the witnesses who had been a patient in a psychiatric hospital. However, most of the early attempts at encouraging the use of psychological principles in the legal system occurred before the field of clinical psychology was formally established and therefore occurred in areas such as perception and cognition (e.g., eyewitness identification). These early attempts were aided by significant figures such as Hugo Munsterberg (Chapter 1) and his book, *On the Witness Stand* (1908), in which he encouraged the use of a variety of psychological findings and methods to aid the court, including some clinically related areas such as criminal behavior. Although his early claims regarding the ability of psychology to make a difference in the courtroom may have been overly optimistic (Benjamin, 2006), Munsterberg did encourage consideration of the possibility despite early critiques by legal scholars such as John Wigmore (see Box 3.1 for discussion of the Wigmore critique of Munsterberg).

The professional status of clinical psychologists in the early part of the twentieth century made it unlikely psychologists would flood courtrooms. During the infancy of clinical psychology, clinical psychologists were largely seen as administrators of psychological tests and certainly secondary to psychiatrists in the mental health field. As a result, psychiatrists were the only ones consistently able to testify in legal matters (Ewing, 2003). This practice changed with *Jenkins v. United States* (1962). The majority opinion in the DC Circuit Court of Appeals, as authored by Judge David Bazelon, whom I will also mention in Chapter 7 (Insanity), reasoned that because of their significant training and expertise, clinical psychologists should not be barred from testifying on mental

Box 3.1.   Discussion of Munsterberg and Wigmore Controversy

Hugo Munsterberg was one of the most eminent psychologists of the early 1900s. He became director of the first psychological laboratory in the United States, originally established at Harvard, and one of the first presidents of the American Psychological Association in 1898. Generally he is recognized not only as the father of forensic psychology but of the entire field of applied psychology.

A figure that was equal to, if not superior, to Munsterberg in his field of the law was John Henry Wigmore. Dean Wigmore was a Harvard educated dean of Northwestern Law School and potentially the most important legal scholar of his time. Wigmore agreed with much of the sentiment Munsterberg expressed in *On the Witness Stand* and had even lectured on such topics as the fallibility of eyewitness testimony before *On the Witness Stand* was published. Nonetheless, Wigmore believed that many of Munsterberg's claims were excessive and without foundation in psychological research. Wigmore carried out his response to Munsterberg in an article in a 1909 issue of the *Illinois Law Review* in a creative fashion. Wigmore framed his response as fictional trial in which a character "Muensterberg" was placed on trial for libeling the legal profession.

Most accounts of the mock trial have alluded to it being similar to other historical events such as Custer's last stand with Munsterberg serving in the role of Custer (Doyle, 2005). Wigmore was able to refute Munsterberg's claims about psychology's application to the law. Though his fictional account left Munsterberg recoiling and some psychological scholars claimed that it left psychology completely disregarded in the eyes of the law (Brigham, 1999), it also provided one of the first opportunities for psychology to learn of the legal community. Moreover, Wigmore is often described as one of the biggest, if not the biggest, proponents of psychology informing the legal system.

health issues, as a matter of law (Ewing, 2003). As Ewing (2003) writes in regard to *Jenkins*, "its importance to the history of forensic psychology cannot be underestimated" (p. 58). Without the decision in *Jenkins*, it is unlikely that we would be experiencing the prolific growth in forensic psychology that has occurred over the past 40 years.

Admissibility of Expert Testimony

In order for psychologists to testify in a trial, their testimony must be legally permissible or admitted by a judge. The admissibility of scientific expert testimony has been of increasing interest over the past decade, as indicated by some significant cases decided by the respective Supreme Courts of the United States and Canada (see *Daubert v. Merrell Dow Pharmaceuticals*, 1993; *Regina v. Mohan*, 1994). However, the admissibility of scientific testimony and psychological testimony can be traced back much further to cases and principles that continue to be relevant today, despite these more recent rulings. It is also extremely important for forensic psychologists to be aware of the legal standards for the admissibility of their testimony because it has a direct bearing on the methods and techniques they utilize in their practice. Even though forensic psychologists are unlikely to testify in the majority of their cases, they must be prepared for the potential in every case.

Frye Standard

In the United States, the relevant standard across most states and the Federal government prior to *Daubert* was the *Frye* standard. In *Frye v. United States* (1923), the DC Circuit Court of Appeals stated that "while courts will go a long way in admitting expert testimony deduced from a well-recognized scientific principle or discovery, the thing from which the deduction is made must be sufficiently established to have gained general acceptance in the particular field it belongs" (p. 1014). Hence, the sole basis for allowing scientific experts to testify under the *Frye* test was that of general acceptance. If a scientific procedure or theory was generally accepted by a particular scientific field, the expert was allowed to testify. If the specific field did not accept the theory or procedure as accurate, the expert was not allowed to testify. For example, in *Frye* the issue was the admissibility of expert testimony regarding a polygraph (i.e., lie detector). The court concluded that the scientific field did not generally accept the polygraph as reliable or valid so such testimony was not admitted into court and polygraph experts continue to be excluded from testifying today. The *Frye* test was easily administered by the courts since it required minimal scientific sophistication from judges (Faigman, Porter, & Saks, 1994).

   The courts also balance the **probative value** of the evidence against the **prejudicial** consequences of admitting the evidence (Taslitz, 1995). The probative value means that a piece of information helps prove a particular point or is useful in deciding an issue before the court. Prejudicial refers to the potential damage or bias a piece of evidence or testimony may cause. All evidence offered in court is both probative and prejudicial. As result, this balancing test means that the information an expert conveys has to be more beneficial (i.e., more probative) than any prejudice or bias that it might introduce into the minds of the judge or jury, the triers of fact, or it will not be admitted into court. For example, past bad acts such as if a defendant murdered someone before are generally not admissible in a criminal trial. The reason is because the courts have determined that this information would bias juries against a defendant unreasonably, it would be too prejudicial, and would provide little, if any, probative value in deciding if the defendant was guilty of the current crime. Expert testimony must meet the same burden of being more beneficial than it is biasing.

Daubert v. Merrell Dow

Many criticized the *Frye* test for only applying to novel or brand new scientific testimony, which meant the courts had trouble defining the appropriate scientific community to decide if it was generally accepted. It also was criticized as too conservative because it excluded reliable evidence that had the misfortune of being novel. Ultimately, the concerns over scientific expert testimony began to focus on the admission of **junk science**. Junk science was considered to be expert testimony admitted on issues that were not well established in the scientific community but were useful to the legal system in some manner. For example, the testimony of representatives of the tobacco companies suggesting that cigarette smoking does not cause cancer has been used as an example of junk science outside of psychology (Givelber & Strickler, 2006). In *Daubert*, the Court concluded that the *Frye* test was obsolete and that the admissibility of scientific expert testimony would now be governed by the requirements of *Daubert* (*Daubert v. Merrell Dow Pharmaceuticals, Inc.*, 1993). See Figure 3.1 for an example of *Daubert* in action.

   Daubert originally involved a claim by two plaintiffs on behalf of their children born with severe birth defects. The trial court excluded the testimony of the plaintiff's experts attempting to prove the link between use of the drug Bendictin and the children's birth defects. The Supreme Court ultimately reversed the lower court decision to exclude the plaintiff's expert evidence and held that the *Frye* general acceptance test was not the proper rule for deciding the admissibility of scientific evidence (*Daubert v. Merrell Dow Pharmaceuticals, Inc.*, 1993). The Court identified the role of the trial judge as that of a gatekeeper in regard to all scientific testimony and specified a two part admissibility screening process that focused upon *relevancy* and *reliability*. The Court indicated that in order for scientific evidence to be relevant, it must relate to the issues at hand. Taking its direction from the relevancy test, the Court indicated that the trial judge had the discretion to exclude relevant testimony when the probative value was outweighed by the prejudicial impact of the testimony.

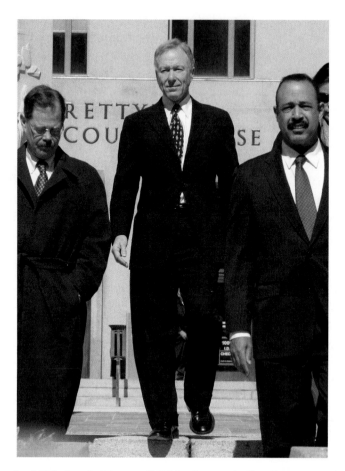

Figure 3.1. In 2005, Lewis "Scooter" Libby Jr. was indicted on numerous charges related to the disclosure of covert CIA agent Valerie Plame. Libby hired several renowned psychologists to present psychological research to jurors but the court deemed the testimony inadmissible under *Daubert* because it believed the underlying studies were of questionable validity; the testimony would not assist the jury; the prejudicial effect of the testimony outweighed its probative value; and the testimony would replace the jury as the trier of fact. © Alex Wong/Getty Images

In devising its second criterion, reliability, the Court relied on Federal Rules of Evidence (FRE) 702 which equates scientific knowledge with reliable expert evidence. However, the court understood the term reliability to mean scientific validity. The Court was incorrect when it suggested that judges were interested in the consistency of expert evidence (reliability) when they were really interested in the accuracy of expert testimony (validity). Nonetheless, to establish reliability the Court identified a list of guidelines:

1. Is the theory or technique at issue testable and has it been tested?
2. Has the theory or technique been subjected to peer review or publication?

need to be aware of the different values of each system and the potential for a resulting loss of their scientific objectivity. Gutheil & Simon (2004) specifically identified several sources of this potential bias in forensic work.

Financial incentives

Maybe the biggest source of a potential bias that leads to the appearance of a corrupt scientific process is the financial reward of serving as an expert. One survey of the case law looking for mentions of *whores* and *prostitutes* directed toward mental health professionals, inspired by the Hagen book, even concluded that "the perception among legal professionals [is] that many mental health experts are unscrupulous" (Mossman, 1999, p. 414). Some experts earn over $10,000 for their work on a single case and there is increasing sensitivity to the appearance and problems associated with being a so called hired gun (Boccaccini & Brodsky, 2002; Cooper & Neuhaus, 2000). Some even suggest there is no such thing as an objective expert anymore and prominent forensic experts have refused to testify in court because of the potential biasing effect (Colbach, 1997). Nonetheless, a survey of attorneys found that the majority of attorneys did not choose forensic psychologists because of their willingness to give a dishonest opinion but based the selection of psychological experts on their knowledge, communication skills, and reputations (Mossman & Kapp, 1998). Forensic psychologists must be very mindful of the perceived bias and make it clear that they are being paid for their time as an expert and not for their testimony.

Extra-forensic relationship

Another issue mentioned by a number of commentators is the occurrence of extra-forensic relationships. These relationships can exist in a number of ways. The most readily identifiable relationships occur when one of the parties involved in a court case is a friend or family member of an expert. However, the extra forensic relationship also can occur when the involved party and the forensic psychologist are members of the same professional organization or institution (Gutheil & Simon, 2004). For example, the forensic psychologist and one of the involved parties could belong to the same civic organization or church. The criticism is that the relationship can cloud the objectivity of the expert and be used to suggest that a given expert's work product or testimony is biased.

Attorney pressure

It is very likely that an expert will feel pressure from attorneys. Attorneys are bound by their own professional ethics to fight for their clients to the best of their ability and they need not be objective in their work. However, the forensic expert is supposed to be honest and objective (Gutheil & Simon, 1999). As a result, it is quite natural for conflict to occur in these situations and for the expert to experience pressure to perform in a certain manner or offer a particular type of testimony. These pressures may come in the form of the attorney expressing an assumed opinion, offering only selective data for the expert's review, claiming to have another expert who will perform the task without any problem, claim financial hardship, or exhibiting an unfavorable response to an initial opinion (Gutheil & Simon, 1999). The expert must be able to identify these instances and resist the pressure to perform in a particular way. In one instance an attorney asked me to delete a reference from my report about a particular psychological test because it was not consistent with the rest of my findings and it was unfavorable for the case. I refused to do so and ultimately the attorney understood my rationale and it was never brought up by the opposing side.

Political and moral beliefs

Another source of potential bias can come from political or moral beliefs (Gutheil & Simon, 2004). Moral biases can arise in cases involving issues like abortion or child custody. Political issues that clash with either side of the conservative and liberal spectrum of political beliefs such as death penalty cases are also problematic for the forensic expert. For example, an expert may choose to only testify for either the prosecution or the defense in these cases because of her beliefs for or against the death penalty. In these instances, the expert's final opinion may be dictated before the evaluation ever takes place and objectivity is completely destroyed. Experts should consider the bias their personal, moral, and political beliefs may introduce and refuse cases in which this bias cannot be properly managed.

Notoriety

Another area of potential bias is because of the limelight or notoriety that may accompany serving as an expert witness (Gutheil & Simon, 2004). Being a part of the media barrage of a given case and receiving public acclaim can be very attractive. A colleague of mine and I have routinely discussed the lure of this type of attention and he has admitted to enjoying aspects of the process. As a result, I have grown fond of referring to him by the name Icarus; from the Greek myth in which Icarus flew too close to the Sun because he lost himself in the thrill of flying. Icarus had a pair of wings made of feathers and wax and they melted as he flew too close to the Sun and he soon crashed to the Earth. In these situations, the forensic psychologist runs the risk of getting too close to the Sun, or the fame of testifying in high profile cases, and may get burned by the loss of objectivity. Although the consequence is not as severe for the forensic psychologist as it was for Icarus, it can still be a source of bias.

Competition

A final source of potential bias is competition (Gutheil & Simon, 2004). Bias from competition may occur for several reasons that relate to the legal context, professionalism, or the expert's personality. For example, an expert might be more prone to take a case, especially a high profile case, which may test her objectivity because another colleague will assist the attorney if she refuses it.

Table 3.2.   Criticisms of Expert Testimony and Sources of Scientific Corruption

1. Taking over the courtroom
2. Testify to the ultimate issue
3. Use of experts corrupts science for several reasons:
    - Financial incentives
    - Extra forensic relationships
    - Attorney pressure
    - Political and moral beliefs
    - Notoriety
    - Competition
    - Lack of a recognition of sources of bias

An expert also may want to perform better than an opposing expert and seek to offer a conclusion not because it is the correct one but because it will trump an opposing expert's opinion. The legal process itself also can encourage tendencies to win that many people, especially successful ones, naturally may have developed over their lifetime. These tendencies may become even greater as an expert becomes more successful testifying, gets more comfortable, and is sought after more frequently by attorneys.

Lack of recognition of bias
However, the real danger in any of these potential sources of bias is not that the bias exists but that the bias goes unrecognized and affects the process, the writing of the report, the conclusion, or even the testimony of the expert (Gutheil & Simon, 2004). At least one study examined potential biases among experts (Commons, Miller, & Gutheil, 2004). Commons et al. (2004) solicited questionnaire responses from 46 attendees at a professional workshop and concluded that experts "wildly underestimate the biasing effects of their own conflicts of interest and other factors" (p. 73). For example, participants did not believe that the amount of money involved in a case, the high profile nature of a case, the expert's personal philosophy or social agenda, or relationship to the attorney hiring them created bias. These results suggest that forensic experts should be especially on guard for sources of potential bias and not minimize the degree to which they may impact their professional judgment. Table 3.2 summarizes the criticisms of expert testimony and sources of scientific corruption.

Ethics of the Expert

An important aspect of performing as a forensic psychologist and especially as an expert witness is adhering to a set of professional guidelines or ethical principles. It is especially important for psychologists in their roles as forensic experts to perform in an ethical manner for many reasons of which we have already touched on in this book. Factors such as the adversarial nature of the legal system, the significant consequences of legal decisions, and the public nature of forensic work all converge to make ethical practice as an expert witness especially important. The legal system sometimes conflicts with the practice of psychology and even the ethical principles of psychologist as objective practitioners of science. The ethical ideal of the adversarial legal system is to fight for a client to the best of your ability, in essence you are not supposed to be objective, you are supposed to be an advocate. As a result, it is even more important that a forensic psychologist maintains a firm ethical foundation in the face of pressure from the legal system. Forensic psychologists assist the legal system with decisions that have far-reaching implications. It is important not only to be correct when testifying on the potential for violence for someone facing the death penalty but to do so in an ethical manner. Also, as discussed in Chapter 1, the public often forms their view of psychology from the media (Stanovich, 2004). The more sensational media images are very likely to come from forensic psychology (Huss & Skovran, 2008). As a result, forensic psychologists have a special duty to behave in an ethical manner because the public forms much of its view of psychology from these media images.

Many professions have a set of ethical principles or ethical guidelines that individuals in that profession follow and psychology is no different. In fact, there are several potential sources of professional and ethical guidelines for forensic psychologists. The primary source of ethical principles for psychologists is the American Psychological Association's Ethical Principles of Psychologists and Code of Conduct (APA, 2002). But why have these ethical codes? Hess (1999) suggests that because society grants a particular profession a monopoly, the profession must take it upon itself to serve the public's best interest and not simply serve the profession. Ethical codes serve these interests. Frankel (1989) identifies several functions for ethical codes that largely focus on the need to educate the public, instill trust in a profession, identify a shared set of values and skills for members of a profession that can serve as a professional compass, and provide a mechanism for sanctions against unethical professionals as well as a mechanism for protecting professionals from unwarranted claims by clients.

Competence

The most obvious area of ethical concern in forensic expert testimony is the need to be competent (Sales & Shuman, 1993). The APA Code (APA, 2002) explicitly states that psychologists should only practice "with populations and in areas only within the boundaries of their competence, based on their education, training, supervised experience, consultation, study or professional experience" (p. 1063). In other words, psychologists must stay within their **scope of practice**. Scope of practice is normally defined as psychologists practicing only in areas in which they are competent. Their competency comes from having sufficient education and experience in a given area to make reliable and valid professional conclusions (Ogloff, 1999). For example, a forensic psychologist is competent to practice forensic psychology but is not competent to practice law unless he or she actually has a law degree and has obtained additional professional experience to practice law. That is not to say that a forensic psychologist does not need to be familiar with the law governing the practice of forensic psychology (Shapiro, 2002) but that the expert must simply avoid practicing as a lawyer instead of a psychologist.

Furthermore, someone might be trained as a forensic psychologist but that does not give her the requisite experience to practice all aspects of forensic psychology. Someone who is only trained to diagnose adult psychopathology would not be competent to perform child custody evaluations. She needs to be familiar with mental illness but also with developmental psychology and the literature on parenting to adequately assess someone in a child custody situation. A psychologist may even be competent to practice in a given area but not competent to use a particular psychological test (Rotgers & Barrett, 1996). A forensic psychologist may attempt to assess someone for depression in a personal injury case but not be competent to use the MCMI-III because he was never trained to do so in graduate school, was never supervised in practice, and never attended any professional workshops on this psychological test (Knapp & VandeCreek, 2001). Furthermore, psychologists have an ethical obligation not only to be competent but to maintain their competence and expertise by participating in opportunities for continuing education. They need to keep up on developments for any method or test they seek to use (Shapiro, 2002).

Scope of practice is not only relevant to individuals practicing within forensic psychology or particular areas of forensic psychology. It is also relevant to the profession as a whole. For example, we will discuss in Chapter 12 not only the relevant legal considerations and psychological techniques involved in child custody decisions but also whether those techniques meet a threshold requirement and are sufficient enough to actually inform the courts. Have we demonstrated adequate reliability and validity to perform child custody evaluations? If not, psychology as whole is practicing outside of its scope of practice. This notion may seem rather simplistic at this point but we will continually discuss instances in which it could be questioned whether forensic psychologists are practicing within their scope of practice.

Informed Consent and Confidentiality

Two other related ethical issues are obtaining informed consent and confidentiality. It is routine in the practice of clinical psychology that we obtain the consent of a client to undergo an evaluation or participate in treatment (Stanley & Galietta, 2006). Informed consent consists of describing the procedures and the process as it is likely to happen and obtaining the client's legal consent to proceed. Obtaining informed consent is also necessary in a forensic context and the APA code of ethics even makes special mention of obtaining informed consent when services are court ordered in 3.10c of the Ethics Code (APA, 2002). In a forensic context, a person may be experiencing additional coercion either because of their own secondary gain or because a legal authority is mandating the evaluation.

Related to obtaining informed consent is the idea of confidentiality. As most people assume, there is both statutory and case law upholding the confidentiality of the therapist–client relationship (Glosoff, Herlihy, & Spence, 2000). Although this privilege does have some limitations depending on the jurisdiction (e.g., reporting child abuse), clients may assume that this privilege exists universally. A problem arises if patients assume this same privilege exists in a forensic assessment because these same privileges of confidentiality are further reduced (Knapp & VandeCreek, 2001). If the court mandates a report or an attorney requests an evaluation of a defendant in a criminal case, the report is going to be read by the judge, the opposing attorneys, and potentially introduced into evidence in open court where the forensic psychologists will testify about it. This practice does not allow for the the same level of confidentiality one normally experiences when seeking therapy.

A problem arises if a forensic psychologist does not explain this limitation to an individual or the individual does not understand this limitation (Hess, 1999). It is important that the examinee recognizes the limits of confidentiality in a given case and that he clearly understood prior to beginning the process. It becomes further complicated because explaining these limitations conflicts with the forensic psychologist obtaining information in an open and honest manner. If a client misunderstands and believes that everything she discusses is confidential, she will be more likely to reveal information that is harmful to her legally and potentially relevant to the evaluation. There is a conflict for the forensic psychologist. On one hand he has an ethical obligation to obtain truly informed consent but on the other hand the assessment will be more accurate if the information he obtains from the parties involved is believed to be confidential. Nonetheless, the ethical responsibility for informed consent is more important.

Financial Arrangements

Another potential ethical issue that experts confront are the financial issues related to being a forensic expert. These issues are increasingly important as forensic psychology is seen as a financially rewarding area of practice (Haas, 1993). This area would seem a rather mundane one for a potential ethical conflict to occur but it is actually of great concern. In fact, the APA Ethical Code (APA, 2002) encourages establishment of financial arrangements as early as possible in the relationship and an expert may even require payment in advance and be very specific about the services being charged for and the specific fees (Knapp & VandeCreek, 2001).

Perhaps the most salient reason for handling financial matters in this manner is the potential impact of any compensation on the forensic conclusion.

Psychologists should not perform forensic services on a **contingency fee** basis where the psychologist is paid for his or her services based on the conclusion (Knapp & VandeCreek, 2006). Such a practice has serious complications for the objectivity of the forensic process. Obvious examples of a contingency fee arrangement are normally easily identifiable but more subtle situations such as an attorney refusing to pay unless a report is "slightly" altered are potentially more dangerous.

Multiple Relationships

The APA Ethics Code (APA, 2002) states that psychologists should avoid multiple relationships "if the multiple relationship could reasonably be expected to impair the psychologist's objectivity, competence, or effectiveness in performing his or her functions as a psychologist, or otherwise risks exploitation or harm to the person with whom the professional relationship exists" (p. 1065). Typically, the focus of multiple relationships as an expert focuses on the conflict between being a treating therapist and acting as a forensic evaluator (Shuman, Greenberg, Heilbrun, & Foote, 1998). There may be situations in which these relationships cannot reasonably be avoided, such as if a psychologist is the only mental health professional in a rural area or a psychologist requires information on a patient who has been court ordered into treatment (Knapp & VandeCreek, 2006). However, the forensic psychologist needs to be aware of the potential harm that can result in these situations.

There are a number of potential ethical problems that can arise from circumstances in which a multiple relationship exists. For example, being asked to evaluate someone in a child custody dispute to whom you have previously delivered psychotherapy (Shapiro, 2002). The difficulty arises because the focus in a forensic context is no longer the welfare of your client but your obligation to the attorney or court that has hired the forensic psychologist. The focus is on giving them objective information (Knapp & VandeCreek, 2006). Suppose a psychologist is treating a woman who is suffering from anxiety and then is asked to perform a custody evaluation to help the court decide the custody of her two children. The psychologist is placed in a potentially compromising situation no matter the conclusion. If the opinion is unfavorable, the finding is very likely to impact the therapeutic relationship in the future and decrease the chances of a successful process because the therapeutic relationship has been damaged. If the conclusion is neutral, the psychologist might be pressured to provide a more favorable conclusion by a client. If the conclusion is positive, there will be an appearance of favoritism. Moreover, a psychologist can never be sure whether his report simply verified his previous therapeutic assumptions or is really objective and truly answers the court's question. As Shapiro (2002) notes, "one cannot be an effective therapist in terms of assisting a client or patient to deal with her or his difficulties if one has been involved in doing a comprehensive forensic evaluation of that individual" (p. 46).

Syndrome Evidence: Controversial Area of Expert Testimony

In concluding the chapter on expert testimony, we will focus on an area of forensic expert testimony that is often controversial. In examining **syndrome evidence** and the controversy that surrounds it, the goal is not to indict forensic psychologists who testify as experts in these cases. In fact, we could choose a variety of other issues such as using psychopathy in death penalty cases or performing risk assessments in Sexually Violent Predator commitment hearings. However, an examination of expert testimony involving syndrome evidence offers a unique opportunity to look at a specific area in which a great deal of controversy exists both from a legal perspective and from a psychological perspective. Syndrome evidence also serves as an example in which psychological information that is useful in one context is questioned, if used in another context. In addition, it helps give a real life context for issues we will be discussing throughout this book, such as staying within one's scope of practice and therapeutic jurisprudence.

Profile and Syndrome Evidence

The use of profile or syndrome evidence has been controversial for decades, almost since their widespread use in psychology and the legal system (Dahir, Richardson, Ginsburg, Gatowski, & Dobbin, 2005; Frazier & Borgida, 1985; Schuller, Wells, Rzepa, & Klippenstine, 2004). For example, Battered Woman Syndrome was first introduced in a United States court in the 1970s (*Ibn-Tamas v. U.S.*, 1979) and later in the Canadian courts (*Regina v. Lavelle*, 1988) in defense of women who killed their abusers. Soon a variety of other syndromes were identified in the psychological literature and made their way into the courts (e.g., Frazier & Borgida, 1985). The terms profile and syndrome have been used interchangeably (Dahir et al., 2005) and will only be differentiated at a superficial level in this discussion. The term syndrome refers to a set of symptoms that occur together in a meaningful manner and typically have a triggering event. Profiles are similar but tend to be more specific and are used to predict behavior because someone matches a particular list of characteristics drawn from the syndrome. For example, many of you have heard of racial profiling in which an individual is identified as someone of interest or arrested largely because of his or her race or ethnicity. If the federal government were to search only those people at the airport who appeared to be of Arab or Muslim decent, it would be using racial profiling. Although racial profiling is one form of profiling, our examination will focus on psychological profiles based on syndromes. The reason we will use these terms interchangeably is that in discussing syndrome evidence, the controversy arises not only from the discussion of the syndrome itself but in experts testifying about syndromes in ways that make them seem more like profiles.

Box 3.2.   Battered Women Syndrome

Battered woman syndrome, as originally conceptualized by Lenore Walker (1979; 1984), consists of a list of characteristics that are subsumed in two primary components, a cycle of violence and application of learned helplessness to women who have been the victims of an abusive partner. Walker stated that women who experienced prolonged abusive relationships often experienced three different phases of violence that included the tension-building phase, the explosion or acute battering incident, and the honeymoon phase that consisted of a calm, loving respite in which the batterer was apologetic for his abuse (Walker, 1979). As a result of this abuse, the woman typically experienced learned helplessness and did not think there was anything she could do to stop the abuse.

The idea of learned helplessness was borrowed from the efforts of Martin Seligman's pioneering work on dogs. Seligman stumbled on the idea of learned helplessness in his research focused on depression. Seligman discovered that dogs who were unable to escape from an apparatus during the delivering of electrical shocks learned to simply lie in the cage when they were later able to avoid the shocks. Walker believed there was a similar principle at work among women who had been the victims of ongoing abusive relationships and resulted in battered woman syndrome. She described four general characteristics of the syndrome that included: (1) the woman believing the violence was her fault; (2) an inability to place the responsibility for the violence with anyone else; (3) fear for her life and the life of her children; and (4) an irrational belief that the abuser is all-knowing and all powerful (Walker, 1984).

There are literally dozens of different syndromes that have been noted in the psychological literature and offered into evidence in the courts (Brodin, 2005). A typical list of syndromes includes battered woman syndrome, rape trauma syndrome, battered child syndrome, child sexual abuse syndrome, child sexual abuse accommodation syndrome, and Munchausen Syndrome by Proxy among others. See Box 3.2 for a fuller description of Battered Woman Syndrome as an example of syndrome evidence. Syndrome evidence was initially used in courts to explain seemingly unusual behavior by someone who was a victim of a specific trauma in order to educate the jury as to the reasonableness of unusual behavior (Moriarity, 2001). Battered woman syndrome would be used to explain the reason for a woman failing to leave an abusive relationship or believing that abuse was imminent despite the batterer being passed out asleep (Huss, Tomkins, Garbin, Schopp, & Kilian, 2006). Rape trauma syndrome would be used as an explanation for a sexual assault victim to continue interacting with her perpetrator in social settings after the assault. Child sexual abuse syndrome would be used to explain the reason for a child failing to report sexual abuse by her stepfather. Syndrome evidence tended to be very helpful for the courts and had both a social and an intuitive appeal when presented by an expert.

However, there were some aspects of this testimony that were unusual. Typically the syndromes were based on the clinical experience of the originators and were not based on extensive research (e.g., see Burgess & Holstrom,

1974 regarding rape trauma syndrome). Furthermore, the research largely failed to validate these syndromes after they were identified by clinicians. For example, the cycle of violence initially explained by Lenore Walker may serve as a useful heuristic to explain the abuse experience for many women but the research has failed to supports its accuracy for decades (see Faigman & Wright, 1997 for a review). Syndromes also are problematic because there are likely to be a significant number of false positives, the number of people who are identified as exhibiting the syndrome who actually do not suffer from it, though they may experience the sexual assault or physical abuse that can trigger the syndrome (Richardson, Ginsburg, Gatowski, & Dobbin, 1995).

However, syndrome evidence is not only being used to explain unusual behavior of a criminal complainant in a sexual assault case or a battered woman who kills her abuser and is charged with a homicide. Syndrome evidence is increasingly used in a substantive manner, directly or indirectly, to support a particular claim with potentially little additional evidence (Moriarity, 2001). **Substantive evidence** is evidence used to prove the fact at issue such as the guilt or innocence of a criminal defendant. For example, a defendant may be charged with sexual assault but admit to consensual sexual intercourse. The burden for the prosecution then becomes not to prove sexual intercourse occurred but that unwanted sexual intercourse occurred. Prosecutors began to call upon expert witnesses to explain that some of the behaviors the victim exhibited were characteristic of a person who suffered from rape trauma syndrome. Their logic followed that the defendant must be guilty of rape because the victim fits the so called profile of someone who has been sexually assaulted. In a slightly different approach, an expert might testify that there are a set of characteristics that are routinely found in domestic violence perpetrators and that a given defendant fits the profile of a domestic violence perpetrator. Even Lenore Walker, the most famous advocate for battered women, was supposed to be called as an expert witness in the O.J. Simpson trial to claim that his ex-wife, Nicole Brown Simpson, did not fit the profile of a battered woman so Mr. Simpson could not have been abusive toward her (Raeder, 1997). Use of syndrome evidence in this manner constitutes **character evidence**. As a rule, character evidence is not admissible unless the defense opens the door by claiming the defendant is of upstanding character. As a result, expert testimony focusing on syndrome evidence has been admitted with less frequency in a substantive manner to prove or disprove a criminal charge.

Syndrome evidence, whether it is battered woman syndrome, rape trauma syndrome or child sexual abuse syndrome, was controversial prior to its use as a substantive claim in criminal trials because of the general lack of empirical support for any of the syndromes. However, substantive expert testimony is especially controversial because syndrome evidence was not intended to be used as a diagnostic tool to determine if a particular abusive act occurred (Allen & Miller, 1995). A sufferer of Munchausen Syndrome by Proxy may exhibit the following symptoms: the primary caregiver of a child, most likely a mother, educated, middle to upper class, highly attentive, friendly with medical staff, takes a child to multiple physicians looking for different medical opinions, and appears calm when presented with difficult news; but that certainly does not mean that anyone who exhibits these behaviors suffers from Munchausen Syndrome by Proxy. This logic suffers from a fundamental flaw. A noted forensic psychologist, John Edens, is fond of this analogy to explain it. Most hard drug users may have started out smoking marijuana but that does not mean that smoking marijuana causes people to then use hard drugs. Almost all hard drugs users started out eating baby food but do you ever hear anyone argue that eating baby food causes hard drug use? Just because someone is a mother, educated, middle class, and highly attentive to her children does not mean she tries to make her children ill and suffers from Munchausen by Proxy.

Legal scholars have claimed that syndrome evidence continues to be successfully admitted despite additional scrutiny because of a host of social, political and legal reasons (Moriarity, 2001). Additional concerns arise that if syndrome evidence continues to be admitted it will lead to a decrease in the rigor and scrutiny that courts use in evaluating scientific evidence. In fact, the Arizona Supreme Court has specifically stated in their admission of syndrome evidence that it was in part admitted because the courts are not equipped to evaluate scientific testimony because of a lack of scientific expertise (Faigman, 2001).

There are significant issues in terms of competent practice and staying within one's scope of practice by testifying in these cases, both for the law and psychology. Psychologists should not use the admissibility of this testimony as a de facto indication that the evidence is of sufficient quality to be used in a psychological context and abdicate their responsibility as scientists. As mentioned in the discussion of *Daubert*, judges are not trained to evaluate this information and make fundamental mistakes in examining syndrome evidence as scientifically sound (Dahir et al., 2005). Expert witnesses also address the ultimate opinion in cases in which syndrome evidence is used to prove or disprove the guilt of a defendant and the accompanying concerns by Melton et al. (1997) and others suddenly appear as a result.

The use of syndrome evidence, especially syndrome evidence used to create a profile and address the substantive legal question, is also a potential example of the anti-therapeutic use of psychology in the legal system. Remember that therapeutic jurisprudence is the legal theory that the law can have both therapeutic consequences (positive consequences broadly speaking) and anti-therapeutic consequences (negative). The potential misapplication of psychological theory by experts and the law is clearly anti-therapeutic if it results in individuals who may require psychological intervention to fail to obtain the assistance or decreases the scientific rigor of expert testimony.

Summary

Since *Jenkins v. United States* (1962) signaled the routine use of the psychologist as an expert witnesses in the United States, the use of forensic experts has grown exponentially. As a result, courts have begun to specify the criteria that expert testimony must fulfill in order to be scientifically sound enough to assist the courts. In the United States, the past standard of general acceptance was *Frye* and this standard has been expanded by the *Daubert* trilogy of cases. Not only has the Court identified more specific criteria to judge experts but the judge has been reaffirmed as the sole gatekeeper and expert testimony need not only be scientific for *Daubert* to apply. Once expert testimony is admitted there are a variety of challenges that face the forensic expert that range from cross-examination to judicial instructions that may contradict the original testimony. However, there also are factors that increase or decrease the credibility of an expert that may serve to buffer or exaggerate those challenges.

Forensic experts have been criticized for taking over the courtroom, offering ultimate opinion testimony, and even corrupting science because of the vast potential for bias. Subsequently, there are a number of ethical responsibilities that forensic psychologists must consider as they testify. Forensic psychologists have a responsibility to be competent and practice within their area of expertise or scope of practice. They must be sure to acquire informed consent and explain the limits of confidentiality despite the difficulty it may pose in the adversarial system. Forensic experts also must be aware of the potential impact of unadvised financial arrangements and multiple relationships on their conclusions. Finally, despite these criticisms and identification of these ethical responsibilities in the literature there are controversial areas of expert testimony, such as the use of syndrome or profile evidence, that may conflict with these ideals and suffer from the criticisms often leveled against forensic experts.

Key Terms

character evidence	meta-analysis	substantive evidence
contingency fee	prejudicial	syndrome evidence
hired gun	probative value	ultimate issue testimony
junk science	scope of practice	

Further Readings

Ewing, C. P. (2003). Expert testimony: Law and practice. In A. M. Goldstein (Ed.), *Handbook of psychology: Vol. 11. Forensic psychology* (pp. 55–66). Hoboken, NJ: John Wiley & Sons.

Gutheil, T. G., & Simon, R. I. (2004). Avoiding bias in expert testimony. *Psychiatric Annals, 34*, 260–270.

PART II Violence and Forensic Psychology

4 Psychopathy

What do you think of when you hear the word **psychopathy**? Does a crazed lunatic, roaming the countryside, committing unspeakable acts and foaming at the mouth come to mind? Do you think of serial killers like Ted Bundy or Jeffrey Dahmer? Unfortunately, these are the images that come to mind for many when they think of a psychopath or the word psychopathy. However, psychopathy encompasses much more than these sensational images. Psychopaths don't just commit some of the most heinous criminal acts we can think of and end up in prison. They may live in the house down the street. They may work in the cubicle next to you or even serve as your elected representative. As Robert Hare's (1999) book stated, even in the title itself (*Without Conscience: The Disturbing World of the Psychopaths Among Us*), psychopaths may truly interact in all aspects of our society. Nonetheless, psychopathy is increasingly relevant to forensic psychology. As Edens (2006) states, "at some point in their careers, clinicians who work or consult in forensic and correctional settings will almost certainly encounter individuals who exhibit psychopathic personality features" (p. 59). Furthermore, Hemphill and Hare (2004) state that psychopathy is the most important clinical construct in the criminal justice system and therefore it is important to any discussion of forensic psychology.

The Nature of the Psychopath

The term psychopathy has a long and varied history that goes back hundreds of years and even has been equated with overall psychopathology or mental illness (Curran & Mallinson, 1944). Millon, Simonsen, Birket-Smith, & Davis (1998) even identify psychopathy as the first personality disorder ever recognized. However, psychopathy is now used to specify a clinical construct or a specific form of **antisocial personality disorder** (APD; Table 4.1) that is prevalent in individuals who commit a variety of criminal acts and generally

Table 4.1.   DSM–IV TR Diagnostic Criteria for Antisocial Personality Disorder

A pervasive pattern of disregard for and violation of the rights of others occurring since age 15, as indicated by three (or more) of the following:

1. failure to conform to social norms with respect to lawful behaviors as indicated by repeatedly performing acts that are grounds for arrest;
2. deceitfulness, as indicated by repeated lying, use of aliases, or conning others for personal profit or pleasure;
3. impulsivity or failure to plan ahead;
4. irritability and aggressiveness, as indicated by repeated physical fights or assaults;
5. reckless disregard for safety of self or others;
6. consistent irresponsibility, as indicated by repeated failure to sustain steady work or honor financial obligations; and
7. lack of remorse, as indicated by being indifferent to or rationalizing having hurt, mistreated, or stolen from another.

behave irresponsibly (Hemphill & Hart, 2003). Robert Hare (1996) has described psychopathy as a socially devastating disorder and that psychopaths are intraspecies predators. However, psychopathy should not simply be equated with criminal behavior (Hare, 2001). Despite the general consensus that psychopathy is related to antisocial behavior there has been a great deal of debate about the criteria and boundaries of psychopathy (Hare, 1996). Some of the debate is apparent in the disagreement about which term best captures the idea we are trying to understand. Is antisocial personality disorder, dyssocial personality, sociopathy, or psychopathy the best term? Part of the debate occurs as we try to identify and understand the true nature of psychopathy.

There is increasing consistency regarding the core traits of psychopathy despite the continued debate over the origin and course of the disorder (Hare, 2001). Hervey Cleckley (1941) was one of the first scholars to offer a comprehensive and definitive conceptualization of psychopathy in his book, *Mask of Sanity*. Cleckley (1941) identified 16 different characteristics that define or compose the clinical profile of the psychopath. The characteristics included: (1) superficial charm and good intelligence; (2) absence of delusions and other signs of irrational thinking; (3) absence of nervousness; (4) unreliability; (5) untruthfulness and insincerity; (6) lack of remorse or shame; (7) inadequately motivated antisocial behavior; (8) poor judgment and failure to learn from experience; (9) pathological egocentricity and incapacity for love; (10) general poverty in major affective reactions; (11) specific loss of insight; (12) unresponsiveness in general interpersonal relations; (13) fantastic and uninviting behavior with drink and sometimes without; (14) suicide rarely carried out; (15) sex life interpersonal, trivial, and poorly integrated; and (16) failure to follow any life plan. Cleckley's (1941) conceptualization was the basis for much of Robert Hare's more recent work (Hare, 1996).

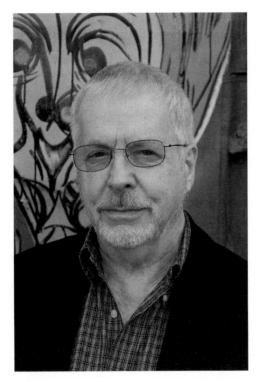

Figure 4.1.   Robert Hare is one of the foremost experts on modern psychopathy and the author of the most frequently used measure of psychopathy, the Psychopathy Checklist-Revised. Photo by Oraf, Vancouver

A Popular Operationalization of Psychopathy: The Psychopathy Checklist

Robert Hare (see Figure 4.1) is often credited as the source of the explosion of research over the past several decades because of his creation of the most widely used measure of psychopathy, the Psychopathy Checklist (PCL) and the current Psychopathy Checklist-Revised (PCL-R). A fundamental problem in the study of the psychopathy until the 1980s was the lack of a standard method for assessing psychopathy, which made it difficult, if not impossible, to compare results across studies (Hare & Neumann, 2006). The PCL and PCL-R gave the field a common description and method for assessing psychopathy. Although the PCL-R is not the only measure of psychopathy, it has become the standard (Huss & Langhinrichsen-Rohling, 2000). Although use of a single measure to define a construct is not without potential problems, the PCL-R is frequently the default measure to assess psychopathy. As a result, the discussion of psychopathy will be largely confined to research using the PCL-R or one of its derivatives such as the Psychopathy Checklist: Screening Version (PCL:SV) and Psychopathy Checklist: Youth Version (PCL:YV).

The PCL-R is composed of 20-items (see Table 4.2) that can be divided into two groups or statistically derived factors. The word checklist is a little bit

Table 4.2. A Comparison of Items on the PCL-R and Cleckley's Characteristics

PCL-R items	Cleckley's characteristics
Overlapping items	
1. Glibness/superficial charm − Factor 1	1. Superficial charm and good intelligence
2. Grandiose sense of self-worth − Factor 1	2. Pathological egocentricity and incapacity for love
3. Pathological lying − Factor 1	3. Untruthfulness and insincerity
4. Lack of remorse or guilt − Factor 1	4. Lack of remorse or shame
5. Shallow affect − Factor 1	5. General poverty in major affective reactions
6. Callous/lack of empathy − Factor 1	6. Unresponsiveness in general interpersonal relations
7. Promiscuous sexual behavior	7. Sex life interpersonal, trivial, and poorly integrated
8. Lack of realistic, long-term goals − Factor 2	8. Failure to follow any life plan
9. Impulsivity − Factor 2	9. Poor judgment and failure to learn from experience
10. Irresponsibility − Factor 2	10. Unreliability
11. Failure to accept responsibility for actions − Factor 1	11. Specific loss of insight
12. Criminal versatility	12. Inadequately motivated antisocial behavior, fantastic and uninviting behavior with drink and sometimes without
Non-overlapping items	
13. Need for stimulation − Factor 2	13. Absence of delusions and other signs of irrational thinking
14. Conning/manipulative − Factor 1	14. Absence of nervousness
15. Parasitic lifestyle − Factor 2	15. Fantastic and uninviting behavior with drink and sometimes without
16. Poor behavioral controls − Factor 2	16. Suicide rarely carried out
17. Early behavioral problems − Factor 2	
18. Many short-term marital relationships	
19. Juvenile delinquency − Factor 2	
20. Revocation of conditional release − Factor 2	

of a misnomer in the name of the PCL-R because it is not simply a list of items that forensic psychologists check off as either being present or absent. A quick look at Table 4.2 and Cleckley's list of psychopathic symptoms suggest several similarities between his original conceptualization and the dominant method for assessing psychopathy. The PCL-R is actually a list of 20 symptoms that requires expert clinical judgment to score. Each item is scored on a 3-point scale ranging from 0 to 2. A score of 0 indicates the absence of a symptom, 1 indicates the possible presence of an item and a 2 is scored if the symptom is definitely exhibited by the examinee. The PCL-R is normally scored through both a review of collateral information and a semi-structured interview. Although the PCL-R can be scored based only on a review of collateral information for research purposes, a clinical interview is recommended, especially for clinical and legal purposes.

Because the PCL-R is scored from 0 to 2 on the 20 items, scores range from 0 to 40 on the measure. A score of 30 and above is considered a conservative cutoff for psychopathy, though some studies have found that scores as low as 25 are appropriate (e.g., Guy & Douglas, 2006). The PCL-R, and psychopathy in general, has been used as a categorical variable, either you are not a psychopath (a score under 30) or you are a psychopath (score of 30 and above). It also has been used as a continuous variable so that the higher the score someone receives, the more psychopathy they exhibit. This distinction has characterized a debate in forensic psychology as to whether psychopathy is best understood on a categorical construct or whether it should be thought of as a continuous score (Edens, Marcus, Lilienfeld, & Poythress, 2006).

Most of the items on the PCL-R are grouped into two categories or factors that were statistically identified as related to psychopathy but separate from one another. These two factors serve as an important distinction for our current understanding of psychopathy. Factor 1 consists of 8 items (as shown on Table 4.2) such as glibness and superficial charm, a grandiose sense of self-worth, pathological lying, as well as others. Factor 1 is often labeled as the interpersonal/affective factor because it is composed of items that largely relate to interpersonal behavior and emotional expression. Factor 2 is often labeled as the socially deviant/antisocial lifestyle factor and consists of behaviorally based items such as parasitic lifestyle, impulsivity, and juvenile delinquency. Three items do not load statistically on either factor, though they are still used to derive a total score on the PCL-R. Recent research also has suggested a three factor model by Cooke and Michie (2001) and a 4 factor-facet model by Hare (2003). However, we will focus on the two factor model for sake of simplicity and because most of the research has been conducted using the two factor approach.

These different categories or factors of psychopathy do not differentiate different types of psychopaths; there are not Factor 1 and Factor 2 psychopaths, though the field is moving toward examining the heterogeneity of psychopathy. One common distinction between different types of psychopathy has been the difference between primary psychopathy and secondary psychopathy. **Primary psychopathy** has been characterized as prototypical psychopathy. The primary psychopath commits antisocial acts, is irresponsible, lacks empathy, and is superficially charming because of some inherent deficit (Skeem, Johansson, Andershed, Kerr, & Louden, 2007). **Secondary psychopathy** in contrast is not inherent but instead caused by "social disadvantage, low intelligence, neurotic anxiety, or other psychopathology" (Newman, MacCoon, Vaughn, & Sadeh, 2005, p. 319). In fact, the key distinction between primary and secondary psychopathy has been the presence of anxiety in the secondary psychopath (Schmitt & Newman, 1999). It has been argued that the secondary psychopath commits antisocial behavior out of impulsivity that is driven by anxiety. It is the absence of any anxiety that has generally characterized the true psychopath and allows him to commit his violence and antisocial behavior repeatedly and without conscience (Levenson, Kiehl, & Fitzpatrick, 1999). However, the difference between primary psychopathy and secondary psychopathy has not been the only issue in need of distinction in regard to psychopathy.

Many students and even psychologists question the difference between psychopathy and the more common term, antisocial personality disorder (APD). Although these two constructs are related and in fact the correlation between psychopathy and APD is large, ranging from .55 to .65 (Hemphill & Hart, 2003), there are also several important differences that distinguish APD from psychopathy (Bodholdt, Richards, & Gacono, 2000).

First, APD is listed in the most widely accepted sources for mental illnesses, the *Diagnostic and Statistical Manual-IV Text Revised* (DSM-IV TR) and in the 10th edition of the *International Classification of Diseases* (ICD-10). Psychopathy is not officially listed in the DSM-IV TR or the ICD-10 as a disorder with the accompanying diagnostic criteria. However, it is mentioned by name under antisocial personality disorder in the DSM-IV TR, the characteristics that compose psychopathy are listed in the associated features of DSM-IV TR, and the term dyssocial personality disorder is used in the ICD-10 to refer to a construct similar to psychopathy (Hemphill & Hart, 2003).

Another difference between APD and psychopathy is related to the diagnostic criteria listed in the DSM-IV TR. The diagnostic criteria for APD are very behavioral (Table 4.2). By behavioral, I mean that DSM tries to increase the reliability of antisocial personality disorder by confining the diagnostic criteria to very objective behaviors such as lying, cheating, and stealing. However, psychopathy is not defined only in behavioral terms, as identified in Factor 2, but also by the interpersonal/affective characteristics that comprise Factor 1. These Factor 1 items may be more difficult to assess than the Factor 2 items. As a result, it is argued that a diagnosis of psychopathy is more narrow and specific than APD.

Accordingly, there are also different prevalence rates for psychopathy and APD. About 3% to 5% of the general public can be diagnosed with antisocial personality disorder and about 50% to 80% of incarcerated offenders. However, only about 1% of the general public suffers from psychopathy and research suggests that only 25% or a range of 15% to 30% of incarcerated offenders are psychopaths (see Figure 4.2). As a result, psychopathy has a much lower prevalence in both the general public and among criminal offenders. APD is often criticized as a diagnosis among offenders because it has little meaning when most offenders can be diagnosed with the disorder. As Bodholt et al. (2000)

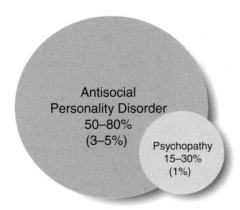

Figure 4.2. The Prevalence and Relationship of Psychopathy and Antisocial Personality Disorder

state, identifying APD "in forensic settings is something like finding ice in your refrigerator" (p. 59). Furthermore, not all people who suffer from psychopathy also suffer from APD. Only about 90% of psychopaths suffer from APD whereas about 15% to 30% of those with APD suffer from psychopathy (Hemphill & Hart, 2003). Individuals who are psychopaths but do not suffer from APD, are often referred to as **successful psychopaths**. Successful or white-collar psychopaths are not incarcerated and tend to exhibit higher intelligence, are more educated, and are from a higher socioeconomic standing than most psychopaths. Successful psychopaths tend to be found working in corporations or holding political office (Hare, 1999). See Box 4.1 for a discussion of successful psychopaths.

The Relationship of Criminal Behavior and Violence to Psychopathy

The distinction between APD and psychopathy is not sufficient to understand the true nature of the psychopath. At the heart of psychopathy is its relationship with criminal behavior, specifically violent criminal behavior. Although there are a number of interpersonal, learning, cognitive, and physiological bases for the expression of violence, it is the violence of the psychopath that routinely captures the imagination of the public and forensic psychologists.

General Violence and Criminal Behavior

Almost since the inception of the PCL-R, its relationship with criminal behavior and violence was explored and the growth in the field is largely a result of this relationship (Edens, 2006). It makes sense that because criminal offenders are most likely to be the subject of studies examining psychopathy that the

Box 4.1. Snakes in Suits: Successful Psychopaths

Nearly all of the research conducted on psychopaths has focused on criminal offenders. The primary reason is that criminal offenders present a captive and easily accessible audience for study. However, non institutionalized studies of psychopaths are nothing new to psychopathy. In fact, one of the earliest studies in psychopathy, prior to the advent of the PCL-R, focused on non institutionalized samples and obtained non institutionalized subjects in a very creative manner. Cathy Widom (1976) placed an ad in the classified section of a Boston newspaper under the guise that she was looking for adventurous people to participate in a psychological study. The ad itself read like a list of the characteristics of psychopaths and resulted in Widom getting almost 30 people to participate whom she identified as potential psychopaths.

Excluding Widom's pioneering study, very few studies have attempted to assess non institutionalized psychopaths outside of college samples. However, Paul Babiak and Robert Hare have begun to examine non institutionalized or successful psychopaths. Specifically, they have pointed to the business world as a source of potential psychopaths and have used the phrase, *snakes in suits* in the title of their recent book, *Snakes in Suits: When Psychopaths Go to Work* (2006). Jobs like used car salesman and politician may be ideal for psychopaths. For example, Michael Douglas's character in the movie *Wallstreet* may be an example of a successful psychopath. However, many of their conclusions about successful psychopaths are not based on empirical studies but are purely anecdotal. Only future research will really tell us whether psychopathic individuals are truly as widespread as they suggest.

focus would often be on the relationship between past and future criminal behavior. It should not be surprising that research has consistently found a relationship between psychopathy and several forms of criminal behavior. In fact, psychopathy has been called the single biggest factor in the assessment of future violence (Salekin, Rogers, & Sewell, 1996) and though not necessary, psychopathy may be sufficient in assessing risk in certain circumstances (Hemphill & Hart, 2003). With the expansion of the study of psychopathy in the past 20 years, there have been an abundance of research studies focusing on the relationship with criminal behavior and several different meta-analyses.

The first meta-analysis examining the relationship between psychopathy and criminal behavior was by Salekin et al. (1996). Studies examining criminal behavior typically use criminal recidivism, or repeat criminal behavior, as an indication of criminal behavior. Salekin et al. (1996) found a significant relationship between psychopathy and general criminal recidivism and an even larger relationship between psychopathy and violent recidivism. Hemphill, Hare, and Wong (1998) took it one step further with a slightly larger group of studies and found a significant but equal relationship with general recidivism and violent recidivism. They found that Factor 2 was a better predictor of general recidivism but that Factor 1 and 2 predicted violent recidivism equally well. Additional meta-analyses have found similar results (Gendreau, Goggin, & Smith, 2003; Walters, 2003b). The available evidence generally suggests that psychopaths are more likely to commit nonviolent crimes and violent crimes than non psychopaths. But what else do we know about the violence of psychopaths compared to non psychopaths?

It is a widely held belief that as we age we are less likely to act out antisocially. In fact, 40 years has often been identified as a threshold age when offenders are likely to "burnout" or show a sharp decrease in their criminal behavior (Huss & Langhinrichsen-Rohling, 2000). This general reduction in crime may be an accurate portrayal of non violent criminal behavior but not violent criminal behavior in psychopaths (Hare, McPherson, & Forth, 1988). Psychopaths appear to continue to commit higher rates of violence than non psychopaths even after the age of 40 (Harris, Rice, & Cormier, 1991). They may even display greater emotional violence (Heilbrun et al., 1998). However, Edens suggests that the available information is not sufficient for forensic psychologists to make definitive conclusions in court concerning the lack of a reduction in violence in psychopaths after age 40 (Edens, 2006; Edens, Petrila, & Buffington-Vollum, 2001).

Another distinction in the violent behavior of psychopaths has been the general nature of their violence. One aspect of psychopathic violence has been the difference between instrumental and reactive violence. **Instrumental violence** is violence that is pursued with a clearly defined goal or is planned and **reactive violence** is perpetrated out of emotion. If you are planning to murder your wife or partner because you want to collect some insurance money, that is instrumental violence. If you come home and find your wife or partner in bed with the mailman and in a fit of anger you pick up the pet rock you have sitting on the dresser and proceed to bash the mailman over the head with it, it would be reactive violence. The belief has long been held that psychopaths are more likely to perpetrate instrumental violence than other non psychopaths or other offenders in general (Cleckley, 1941). More current research has largely validated these theoretical beliefs. Williamson, Hare, and Wong (1987) found that psychopaths were more likely to perpetrate instrumental violence than non psychopathic offenders and less likely to have experienced emotional arousal in a Canadian sample of offenders. Cornell et al. (1996) verified these results among U.S. prisoners. In addition, Cornell et al. (1996) concluded that psychopaths are able to inflict serious injury for goal-directed purposes because of their lack of well-socialized norms, guilt, and remorse.

Nonetheless, the relationship between psychopathy and instrumental violence is not completely clear because psychopaths also exhibit several symptoms such as poor behavioral controls that suggest they are more likely to commit reactive or impulsive violence. Even though Williamson et al. (1987) found that psychopaths were significantly more likely to commit instrumental violence than non psychopaths (42.5% compared to 14.6% of the time), the majority of their violence was reactive. In fact, Hart and Dempster (1997) referred to psychopathic violence as impulsively instrumental. Woodworth & Porter (2002) found that Factor 1 scores but not Factor 2 scores were related to instrumental violence. Therefore it may be that Factor 2, antisocial and deviant features of psychopathy, predicts violence but Factor 1 predicts the nature of the violence and whether it is reactive or instrumental (Porter & Woodworth, 2006).

A number of other features also may distinguish psychopathic violence. Psychopaths are more likely to victimize strangers than are non psychopaths (Hare, McPherson et al., 1988). Williamson et al. (1987) found in their study that none of the murders committed by psychopaths involved family members compared to 63% of murders among non psychopaths. Violence committed by psychopaths is more likely to occur out of revenge and rarely in self-defense (Hart, 1998), which is probably related to the increased likelihood of instrumental violence. Psychopaths' most serious violence is likely to occur during intoxication because they fail to maintain their emotional control when under the influence of alcohol or drugs (Hare, McPherson et al.). A surprising finding is that although psychopaths are more likely to inflict more severe violence than non psychopaths, they are less likely to murder (Williamson et al.). This finding may occur because murders often result out of an emotionally charged situation and are therefore uncharacteristic of psychopaths (Williamson et al.). Woodworth and Porter (2002) further found that when psychopaths do commit murder it is more likely to involve instrumental characteristics (93.3%) than reactive and that they are almost twice as likely as non psychopaths (48.4%) to perpetrate a murder that is largely instrumental.

The literature is very clear that psychopathy plays a unique role in the expression of violence. Although psychopaths may only constitute 25% of criminal offenders they may account for a disproportionate amount of the violence committed (Huss & Langhinrichsen-Rohling, 2000). Psychopathic violence may have several important characteristics that make it especially problematic and unique compared to most violence. However, the link between psychopathy and the commission of criminal behavior and violence is not simply limited to general offenders but also has been examined in other types of criminal behavior.

Sexual Violence

Although Cleckley (1941) has little to say about the role of sexual aggression in psychopaths, their sexual promiscuity and lack of emotional responsiveness in interpersonal relationships may suggest increased risk for sexual violence. Several studies have found that psychopathy is predictive of sexual recidivism among rapists and child molesters and related to sexual arousal in general (Quinsey, Rice, & Harris, 1995; Rice & Harris, 1997; Rice, Harris, & Quinsey, 1990). In fact, offenders with higher scores on the PCL-R commit more frequent and more severe levels of violent sexual offenses (Gretton, McBride, Hare, O'Shaughnessy, & Kumka, 2001). Although the frequency of psychopathy ranges from 15% to 30% among general offenders, about 10% to 15% of child molesters and 40% to 50% of rapists are probably also psychopaths (Brown

& Forth, 1997; Porter, Fairweather, Drugge, Hervé, & Birt, 2000; Quinsey et al. 1995). As these statistics suggest, there are differences among sex offenders.

Generally sexual offenders can be divided into those who perpetrate sexual violence against adults (rapists), children (child molesters), and both children and adults (mixed). Knight and Guay (2006) concluded in their review of the literature that psychopaths are more likely to commit rape and are overrepresented in samples of rapists. Quinsey et al. (1995) found a higher prevalence of psychopathy in rapists than child molesters. Porter, Campbell, Woodworth, and Birt (2001) found that rapists and mixed group offenders had higher scores on the PCL-R than child molesters and that offenders who sexually victimized both children and adults were as high as ten times more likely than other offenders to be psychopaths (Porter, Campbell, Woodworth, & Birt., 2002). Porter et al. (2000) also found that mixed rapist/molesters had the highest Factor 1 scores, suggesting an increased level of insensitivity and callousness. In fact most offenders who perpetrate on both children and adults are psychopathic (Rice & Harris, 1997). Porter et al. (2000) even suggested a distinct category of sexual offenders, sexual psychopaths.

Violence in Civil Psychiatric Patients

It makes sense that psychopathy is important in the expression of violence among general offenders and sex offenders but what about a population in which the expression of violence is not as high? As we will discuss in Chapter 9, an individual who is found to be mentally ill and dangerous may be hospitalized via civil commitment in order to protect others from any potential violence. Nonetheless, the risk of violence among civil psychiatric patients is much lower than general offenders and the importance of psychopathy among civil psychiatric patients is less obvious. Skeem & Mulvey (2001) conducted one of the early examinations of psychopathy in a sample of civil psychiatric patients. They found that even in this less violent sample that psychopathy was a strong predictor of violence. The importance of psychopathy as a predictor of violence in civil psychiatric samples as been duplicated in other studies (Douglas, Ogloff, Nicholls, & Grant, 1999; Nicholls, Ogloff, & Douglas, 2004).

Violence Among Domestic Violence Perpetrators

Domestic violence is another type of violence that has been examined for a potential relationship with psychopathy. Although the perpetration of domestic violence has often been associated with societal and cultural reasons for violence, some have suggested an important role for psychopathy (Huss, Covell, & Langhinrichsen-Rohling, 2006; Spidel, et al., 2007). Recent studies have examined the presence of psychopathy among criminal offenders with domestic violence histories (Grann & Wedin, 2002; Hilton, Harris, & Rice, 2001). Results from both studies suggest that psychopathy is a useful construct in predicting future violence among offenders with a history of domestic violence. However, these studies did not examine domestic violence per se but offenders who had committed domestic violence as one of potentially many crimes. Huss and Langhinrichsen-Rohling (2006) examined psychopathy in a clinical sample of batterers referred for domestic violence treatment and found little predictive relationship between psychopathy and domestic violence above antisocial behavior. As a result, the relationship between psychopathy and domestic violence is less clear than for other types of violence.

What Else Do We Know about Psychopathy?

It is also important to remember that though psychopathy may be the most robust predictor of violence across a variety of types of violence, the PCL-R is not intended to be a risk assessment measure. In Chapter 5, we will examine measures designed specifically to assess the likelihood of future violence. The PCL-R is not one of these tools but is a diagnostic tool for psychopathy (Hart, 1998). Psychopathy just happens to be a good predictor of violence. In addition to the violence and criminal behavior associated with psychopaths, we also have accumulated a great deal of information about how and why psychopaths behave the way they do. Some of this information is similar to Cleckley's original conceptualization but much of it explains some of their potentially contrasting behavior that was simply a mystery before. Even though the information is less applied than the discussion so far, it is still important for forensic psychologists to be aware of this research in attempting explain psychopathic behavior.

Interpersonal/Affective Aspects of Psychopathy

By examining the list of Factor 1 items, it is easy to understand that interpersonal and emotional deficits are central to understanding psychopathy. Characteristics such as glibness and superficial charm, a grandiose sense of self-worth, pathological lying, conning and manipulativeness, lack of remorse and guilt, shallow affect, callous lack of empathy, and failure to accept responsibility for one's actions are going to play a significant role in one's ability to interact and maintain relationships with other people. Psychopaths may be great to introduce at a party or act as a media spokesperson for a product advertisement. However, you would not want to have to count on a psychopath to come pick you up after your car breaks down, try to get across to him your despair after not getting into graduate school, and you certainly would not want to marry one. These interpersonal and affective deficits impede the psychopaths' ability to interact long-term with all other humans.

One of the striking features of psychopaths is their altered emotional or affective responses in their language (Hiatt & Newman, 2006). Psychopaths

Box 4.2.   Careful What You Wish for in the Treatment for Psychopaths

Rice et al.'s 1992 study is one of the most often cited studies on psychopathy. In fact, it was referenced, though incorrectly, repeatedly in the final season of the television show, *The Sopranos*, as proof that psychopaths get worse in therapy. In their study, Rice and colleagues found that 22% of the non psychopaths who were treated violently recidivated after they were released compared to 39% of the untreated non psychopaths. This outcome was certainly expected. One would hope that treatment is effective. However, their findings regarding psychopaths were quite surprising and have been heralded ever since as an indication that treating psychopaths is a much different matter. They found that 55% of the untreated psychopaths violently recidivated but that 77% of the treated psychopaths became violent after they were released. It was not just that treatment did not work but that the treatment made them worse! This study was immediately heralded as evidence to support the long held notion that psychopaths do not respond to conventional psychological treatment.

However, the problem was that the treatment was anything but conventional. The treatment unit where these offenders were being held employed a fairly unconventional form of treatment called *defense disrupting therapy*. The treatment tended to be very intense. More interesting though was that it included nude encounter sessions that lasted as long as two weeks. Staff also forced offenders to use drugs such as LSD and alcohol during treatment sessions (D'Silva et al., 2004). Obviously, generalizing the results of such an unconventional treatment to all treatment of psychopaths is problematic.

criticized for the over inclusiveness of studies in his meta-analysis, especially studies that did not use the PCL-R as the measure of psychopathy (Harris & Rice, 2006). Others have said that there is not sufficient evidence to support either contention that treatment is effective or ineffective for psychopaths (Edens, 2006; Harris & Rice, 2006) but a systematic review arrived at the same conclusion as Salekin, focusing on treatment studies only using the PCL-R (D'Silva, Duggan, & McCarthy, 2004). Nonetheless, there may be some hope for the future as several experts have identified important components to the treatment of psychopathy (Huss, Covell et al., 2006; Losel, 1998; Wallace, Vitale, & Newman, 1999).

Special Groups and Psychopathy

In reviewing the major issues related to psychopathy, one thing should be clear. The research focusing on violence, interpersonal/affective deficits, cognitive/ learning deficits, and treatment has largely been based on a narrow group of psychopaths. The studies have largely been conducted using institutionalized, adult, Caucasian men from Canada and the United States. As a result, a scope of practice question arises. In what other groups is it appropriate to use the PCL-R or use psychopathy as an important factor is assessing risk? In this section I discuss some of the research regarding psychopathy in more diverse groups in order to get a more comprehensive view of the extent of psychopathy.

Women

Although Cleckley (1941) originally included women in his discussion of psychopathy, women have been largely ignored in the study of psychopathy. As their presence in our jails and prisons grows, the role of psychopathy among them has been increasingly examined. The study of psychopathy among women is especially important because of the consistent finding that there are significant differences in the prevalence and expression of externalizing (substance abuse, antisocial personality disorder) and internalizing (depression, anxiety) disorders between men and women (Robins & Regier, 1991). As a result, researchers have begun to examine the prevalence, behavioral manifestations, and clinical correlates of psychopathy in women and found some similarities but also some differences with their male counterparts.

Reviews of the literature on women and psychopathy have generally found lower prevalence rates than with men (Vitale & Newman, 2001). The lower prevalence rates should not be surprising since this finding is consistent with the prevalence of disorders like antisocial personality disorder and conduct disorder. As discussed before, the prevalence rates of psychopathy in incarcerated men range from 15% to 30% but 25% is typical. Women exhibit similar though more varied levels (Verona & Vitale, 2006). Studies have found prevalence rates higher than 30% (Louth, Hare, & Linden, 1998) and as low as 9% (Vitale, Smith, Brinkley, & Newman, 2002). Not only has research found that fewer women score above the traditional cutoff of 30 but that women also exhibit lower mean scores on measures of psychopathy than men (Alterman, Cacciola, & Rutherford, 1993; Rutherford, Cacciola, Alterman, & McKay, 1996).

There also appear to be differences in the behavioral manifestations of psychopathy in women. The relationship between psychopathy and aggression is very clear in male psychopaths. However, the findings for women are not as clear. There have been several studies that have found a relationship between past violent and non violent convictions, self-reported violence, and past arrests in women (Vitale et al., 2002; Weiler & Widom, 1996). When Salekin, Rogers, Ustad, and Sewell (1998) focused on the relationship of psychopathy and future recidivism in women, they found only a moderate relationship, at best, and concluded that only Factor 1 of the PCL-R was related to recidivism. Verona and Vitale (2006) suggest that these inconsistent findings may be because of the differences found in the development of aggression in boys and girls from a young age.

Another important consideration in the examination of psychopathy among women is the underlying clinical presentation of the disorder. Men and women are likely to exhibit certain symptoms in different ways. For example, in terms of violence a male psychopath may get into a bar fight whereas a female psychopath may be more likely to be violent toward family members and in her own home (see Robbins, Monahan, & Silver, 2003). It may well be that they both have underlying predispositions towards antisocial behavior but that these dispositions are expressed in different ways. In fact, Lilienfeld and colleagues (Cale & Lilienfeld, 2002; Lilienfeld, 1992; Lilienfeld & Hess, 2001) suggest that disorders such as borderline personality disorder, somatization disorders, and histrionic personality disorder may be female expressions of psychopathy because of the significant overlap in these disorders and antisocial behavior. For example, Verona and Vitale (2006) use the movie *Fatal Attraction* and Glen Close's character as a possible example of this manifestation. In the movie, Glen Close's character is obsessed with Michael Douglas' character to the point of extreme violence. In addition, she is manipulative, conning, impulsive, lacks empathy and remorse for her behavior that is intended to prevent him from ending their affair and returning to his wife and family. Angelina Jolie's character in *Girl Interrupted* might be another fictional example with similar characteristics. The behavior of either of these two characters is often characterized as indicating borderline personality disorder but it may be that women are more likely to express psychopathic features in this way because of the difference in externalizing versus internalizing behaviors between men and women.

Ethnic and Cross-Cultural Issues

As we became more confident of the nature of psychopathy in Caucasian samples in North America, attention began to turn toward the cross-cultural and multicultural extensions of psychopathy. Hare (2003) has concluded that the PCL-R is generally appropriate to use with a variety of ethnicities and nationalities. However, there are some limitations and differences in assessing psychopathy outside the foundation for most of the research.

One of the first questions regarding the generalization of psychopathy was its applicability to African-Americans, despite their overrepresentation in correctional facilities across the United States. Early efforts at using the PCL-R often excluded African-Americans (Kosson & Newman, 1986) because of the lack of reliability and validity of the PCL-R for African-American offenders. Kosson, Smith, and Newman (1990) conducted a series of studies in which African-American's were included and found the scores of African-American offenders slightly elevated in comparison to Caucasian offenders. However, additional studies have not found the same results consistently (see Sullivan & Kosson, 2006, for a review).

Skeem, Edens, Camp, and Colwell (2004) conducted a meta-analysis to resolve these discrepancies and found that there were differences in total score but that there were not differences in Factors 1 and 2 of the two-factor model of psychopathy. Skeem et al. (2004) concluded there was not sufficient evidence that African-American's have higher core psychopathy traits than Caucasians. Although they believe that psychopathy can be measured reliably and in a valid manner in African-Americans, Sullivan & Kosson (2006) disagree with Skeem et al. and suggest that future research should examine ethnic differences more closely. Furthermore, research should not only examine differences between African-Americans and Caucasians but also other understudied ethnic groups.

In addition to ethnic differences, psychopathy also has been studied cross-culturally. Although the PCL-R has largely been used on offenders in Canada and the United States, there are a number of published studies in countries such as Scotland, England, Belgium, Norway, Spain, Portugal, the Netherlands, Germany, Argentina, and Sweden (see Sullivan & Kosson, 2006). Despite the widespread use of the PCL-R, examination of cross-cultural differences have been recent and data for Great Britain and Sweden only appeared in the most recent PCL-R manual (Hare, 2003). Furthermore, most of the research has focused on comparing European (even largely British) samples with North American samples. As a result, any conclusions that can be made about the cross-cultural application of psychopathy are tentative.

Nonetheless, there appears to be some important cross-cultural differences in psychopathy. Overall, the prevalence and mean scores appear to be higher in the North American samples. Sullivan and Kosson (2006) compared the mean score across offenders, psychiatric patients and forensic patients for 19 samples outside of North America and compared their average score of 18.7 to an average score of 22.1 in the PCL-R manual. As a result of the differences between North American and Scottish samples, Cooke and Michie (1999) recommended using a cutoff score of 25 for psychopathy in Scotland, instead of 30. Other European psychologists have also adopted this modified cutoff score. Nonetheless, psychopathy appears to be a robust predictor of violent and general recidivism cross-culturally (Hare, Clark, Grann, & Thorton, 2000; Tengström, Grann, Långstrom, & Kullgren, 2000) and the cognitive and emotional deficits appear to be present across different countries (Pastors, Moltó, Vila, & Lang, 2003; Pham, Vanderstukken, Philippot, & Vanderlinden, 2003). Though there may be cross-cultural differences in psychopathy, it is equally as clear that psychopathy remains a valid construct with application outside of North America (Sullivan & Kosson, 2006).

Children and Adolescents

In addition to examining the generalizability of psychopathy to a more diverse group of adult offenders, research also has focused on psychopathy in children and adolescents. The first major problem with extending psychopathy to children and adolescents is the same one that plagued the field prior to the 1980s, measurement. The most often used measure of psychopathy in adults, the PCL-R, is not applicable to youth. For example, items like many short-term marital relationships and adult criminal versatility are not going to apply to youth. As a result, early studies focusing on youth used a modified version of the PCL-R that became known as the Psychopathy Checklist: Youth Version (PCL:YV). Several items on the PCL:YV were replaced and altered in order to be applicable to youth and specifically it is intended for use with youth 13 to 18 years of age (Forth, Kosson, & Hare, 2003). Two additional measures of psychopathy, the Antisocial Process Screening Device (ASPD) and the Childhood Psychopathy Scale (CPS), were designed to assess children as young as 6 years-old (Salekin, 2006). Preliminary research has revealed that there is some support for the two factor model originally found in adults but that there may be some slight differences in the items that load on the respective factors in youth (Forth, 1995; Frick, Bodin, & Barry, 2000).

As with adults, one of the initial areas of interest was violence and antisocial behavior. There are a number of studies examining psychopathy in youth and the relationship with antisocial behavior, with consistent results. Studies have found that youth who score high in psychopathy perpetrate more antisocial behavior (Corrado, Vincent, Hart, & Cohen, 2004) and they commit more severe violence (Gretton, Hare, & Catchpole, 2004). Results suggest that youths with psychopathic characteristics exhibit a similar relationship to violence and antisocial behavior as do adults. Recently, Lynam, Caspi, Moffitt, Loeber, and Stouthamer-Loeber (2007) conducted the first study examining the long-term stability of psychopathy and found some evidence for the stability of psychopathy from adolescence to adulthood.

However, there is much less consensus and evidence for the extension of some of the cognitive and emotional aspects of adult psychopathy within youth. Vitale et al. (2005) found expected differences in a Stroop-like task but only found evidence of passive avoidance learning in boys. Roussy and Toupin (2000) also found evidence of deficits in cognitive tasks designed to assess specific regions of the frontal lobe for which adult psychopaths have shown consistent characteristic performance patterns. In addition, other studies have supported the notion that children with psychopathic features have difficulty with automatic processing (O'Brien & Frick, 1996), an inclination for sensation seeking (Frick, O'Brien, Wooton, & McBurnett, 1994), and impulsivity deficits (Blair, 1999).

Even if psychopathy is a valid construct for youth, there is a great deal of debate about the appropriateness of the psychopathy label in children. Much of the debate focuses on the fact that childhood and adolescence is a time of enormous developmental change and that for some youths this change includes acting out in an antisocial manner (Moffit, 1993). As a result, it is very difficult to measure constructs like impulsivity and irresponsibility when these behaviors are likely to change and may even be encouraged in children (Edens, Skeem, Cruise, & Cauffman, 2001). Moreover, a label of psychopathy may have profound implications in the classroom or the legal system (Edens, Guy, & Fernandez, 2003). Some have encouraged the use of other terms rather than psychopathy (Johnstone & Cooke, 2004). Nonetheless, there are many reasons to be cautious with the application of psychopathy to children and adolescence, regardless of the sufficiency of the research.

Legal and Ethical Issues Involving Psychopathy

Psychopathy is used in a variety of legal contexts and Edens and Petrila (2006) even go so far as saying that psychopathy "is becoming pervasive in the law" as "it is increasingly being found in both judicial opinions and legislation, and it also has been the focus of expert testimony" (p. 573). Though an abstract notion of psychopathy has a legal history that dates back almost 100 years, it is only more recently that the term or a variation has been used explicitly (Reed, 1996). Lyon and Ogloff (2000) searched the appellate case law and found that psychopathy was used in a variety of cases including areas such as the death penalty, insanity, competency to stand trial, child custody, the credibility of witness, transfer of juveniles to adult courts, civil commitment, and civil torts. DeMatteo and Edens (2006), in a comprehensive review of the available U.S. case law, found that there have been recent sharp increases in the admission of the PCL-R. However, even though the term has become widely used in the legal system, the legal notion of psychopathy does not always match the clinical or the psychological notion. For example, the term sexual psychopath is being increasingly used in the law to mean someone who fails to maintain control over his sexual impulses (Mercado, Schopp, & Bornstein, 2005) but a lack of control is not the defining feature of psychopathy. Therefore, if a forensic psychologist uses the PCL-R while evaluating a sexual offender the results may be useful clinically to determine whether the individual can be diagnosed as a psychopath. However, a score of 30 and above on the PCL-R does not mimic the legal definition of psychopathy and may be a reason for concern in offering this type of information to the courts (Edens & Petrila, 2006).

Capital Sentencing and the Use of Psychopathy

As with the other issues in this book, psychopathy has relevance for two terms previously introduced, therapeutic jurisprudence and scope of practice. Although, capital sentencing decisions do not represent the most prevalent types of evaluations in which psychopathy is used (DeMatteo & Edens, 2006), they do provide an excellent situation to examine both the impact of the law and the potential limits of expert testimony.

The United States Supreme Court has held that there must be limitations on eligibility to receive the death penalty in capital cases and that specific characteristics of the accused are relevant in that determination (Hesseltine, 1995). A forensic psychologist is often called to testify in the sentencing phase of these trials, after the accused has been determined guilty, in order to determine the individual's risk for future violence. Though commentators have identified a host of problems with expert testimony in capital sentencing decisions (Cunningham & Reidy, 1999), there are also specific problems with employing psychopathy as a potential issue. A forensic psychologist called to testify in these instances will typically offer testimony as to the defendant's risk for future violence to assist the court in determining whether life in prison or the death penalty is the most appropriate sentence. If an individual is at significant risk for violence or even murder while serving life in prison, the court may determine that the death penalty is the most appropriate sentence to protect other inmates and correctional staff.

Experts have testified in these instances that the defendant poses substantial risk if sentenced to life in prison because he scores above the cutoff score of 30 on the PCL-R (Edens, 2001). Given the extensive literature supporting the notion that psychopathy is potentially the best predictor of future violence (Salekin et al. 1996), this conclusion does not initially seem problematic. However, the problem is that the literature examining the potential predictive effect of psychopathy for future violence has largely focused on community violence. The research has focused on the likelihood of psychopaths engaging in violence when left unsupervised in the community. This situation is not the same for a person who is sentenced to life in prison. Not only is such a person incarcerated but that person may be locked down 23 hours per day for the rest of his life. Nonetheless, one of the first studies examining the association between psychopathy and violence during incarceration found a significant correlation between institutional violence and psychopathy (Forth, Hart, & Hare, 1990). However, most reviews of the literature have concluded that there is a non-significant to modest relationship between any institutional misconduct and psychopathy. Cunningham and Reidy (1999) went further and concluded that there was virtually no empirical evidence supporting the use of the PCL-R in death penalty cases where the individual was not only institutionalized but locked down in a high security prison. A recent meta-analysis by Guy, Edens, Anthony, and Douglas (2005) supported these reviews and found only a small correlation of .11 between psychopathy and physical violence.

As this evidence suggests, one could argue it is outside a forensic psychologist's scope of practice to testify that based on a diagnosis of psychopathy a convicted murderer should be sentenced to death. Several scholars have argued that the research does not support a claim for this link regarding institutional violence and that it is even more difficult to support such a link given the lower rates of institutional violence for offenders serving life sentences (e.g., Edens, Buffington-Vollum, Keilen, Roskamp, & Anthony, 2005). The research does not offer the forensic psychologist any expertise in making competent conclusions in these situations to date. However, others point out the significant relationship between psychopathy and almost every other form of violence and suggest that psychopathy is relevant to these determinations and maybe even necessary.

Additionally troubling may be that the profound impact that a label of psychopathy carries. Edens, Colwell, Desforges, & Fernandez (2005) found that when an expert testified that a defendant was psychopathic, a much greater percentage of jurors supported the death sentence. As a result, the legal system is faced not only with imposing the most severe consequence possible, the death penalty, but in doing so based on expert testimony that is not generally supported by the literature. Although some may question the therapeutic nature of the death penalty in general, the current focus has nothing to do with the overall issue of the death penalty. The anti-therapeutic implications of admitting expert testimony that is not supported by research on any issue is clear. The implications become even more profound if different jurisdictions begin to specifically mention psychopathy as an aggravating factor in death penalty cases similar to statutes in Canada that have done so in regard to non capital cases (Zinger & Forth, 1998).

Summary

Psychopathy has long been of interest to forensic psychologists but it is only since the arrival of a common conceptualization and a standard measure that a clearer understanding of the disorder has occurred. The advent of the PCL-R has led to an explosion of research on psychopathy. This research has identified underlying factors that add to our understanding of psychopathy and serve as a basis for differentiating psychopathy from antisocial personality disorder. In addition to the significance of Factor 1 in differentiating psychopathy and APD, the lower prevalence and formal presence of psychopathy in the DSM also differentiate the two constructs.

A host of differences between psychopaths and non psychopaths have become evident across a number of dimensions. The most widely studied aspect of psychopathy has been its relationship to criminal behavior. Not only does psychopathy appear to exhibit a significant relationship with general criminal behavior and violent recidivism but it does so in a variety of individuals at risk to perpetrate future violence. It is also clear that there are unique characteristics of the violence committed by psychopaths. The literature has become clearer regarding the interpersonal, cognitive, and physiological manifestation of psychopathy as they relate to the constellation of psychopathic characteristics and the violence associated with psychopaths.

Despite the fact that much of the research has focused on Caucasian, male, adult offenders in Canada and the United States, there also appears to be an application for psychopathy across a variety of individuals such as women, children and other ethnicities and nationalities. Psychopathy is a valid construct in women although there are reduced prevalence rates among women and the relationship to violence is not as strong. Evidence also exists that psychopathy can be diagnosed in children and adolescents, although some question the appropriateness of the diagnosis. The importance of psychopathy is even supported among a variety of ethnicities and cultures. Nonetheless, forensic psychologists should be aware of the potential differences among diverse groups just as they should be aware of the ramifications of using psychopathy in certain legal contexts such as capital sentencing decisions.

Key Terms

antisocial personality disorder
instrumental violence
passive avoidance learning
primary psychopathy
psychopathy

reactive violence
secondary psychopathy
sham emotions
successful psychopaths

Further Readings

Babiak, P., & Hare, R. D. (2006). *Snakes in suits: When psychopaths go to work.* New York: Regan Books/HarperCollins Publishers.
Hare, R. D. (1999). *Without conscience: The disturbing world of the psychopaths among us.* New York: Guilford.

Box 5.1.   Experts Cannot Predict Violence, So What!
Barefoot v. Estelle (1983)

The most important single case in the history of risk assessment involved Thomas Barefoot, largely because it surprised forensic psychology by encouraging the continued practice of violence risk assessments. Thomas Barefoot burned down a bar in Texas and then later shot the police officer investigating the arson. In 1978, he was convicted of murder and awaited sentencing. One of the questions before the court during the sentencing hearing was the probability of Barefoot being violent again and continuing to be a threat to society (*Barefoot v. Estelle*, 1983). During the sentencing hearing, one psychiatrist, Dr James Grigson, testified there was 100% absolute certainty that Barefoot would commit future violence in prison, if he was not executed. Grigson further stated that Barefoot was above a 10 on a 1 to 10 point scale of sociopathy. In addition, this psychiatrist and another expert testified for the state without ever interviewing the defendant, a significant professional error (Cunningham & Goldstein, 2003; Litwack et al., 2006). Dr Grigson was later expelled from the American Psychiatric Association (Cunningham & Goldstein, 2003) but did not lose his license and continued to practice psychiatry for decades.

On appeal, Barefoot challenged the testimony of the psychiatrists. The American Psychiatric Association filed an **amicus curiae** brief. An amicus brief is a legal document written by a person or entity that is not a party in a given case but has an interest in the matter before the court. An amicus brief is used to inform the court of relevant considerations in which the interested party has some special expertise. The American Psychiatric Association questioned the validity of opinions on future dangerousness and pointed to literature that predictions of future dangerousness were unreliable, given they were inaccurate two out of every three times. The Court agreed that this type of testimony was not always correct but believed that the adversarial process would be able to properly screen it and that juries would assign it the appropriate weight.

too arbitrary and inaccurate. The Court specifically stated that, "from a legal point of view there is nothing inherently unattainable about a prediction of future criminal conduct" (p. 278). More recent cases concerned with the confinement of sex offenders for civil commitment have only solidified the use of expert testimony for predictions of future violence (*Kansas v. Crane*, 2002; *Kansas v. Hendricks*, 1997). Although they did not focus on the admissibility of expert testimony itself, there are additional Supreme Court decisions that required a finding of dangerousness that are equally important to the advancement of risk assessment. *O'Connor v. Donaldson* (1975) demanded that the criteria in civil commitment include dangerousness and by doing so led the courts to seek out expert opinions on future dangerousness. *Tarasoff v. Regents of the University of California* (1976) required practicing mental health professionals, not just forensic psychologists, to exhibit a duty to protect individuals at risk for becoming victims of future violence and thereby they must assess for future

Table 5.1. Important Legal Cases in the Development of Risk Assessment

Supreme Court case	Relevant aspects of the decision
O'Connor v. Donaldson (1975)	A person cannot be committed only on the basis of a mental illness but must also exhibit imminent dangerousness
Tarasoff v. Regents of the University of California (1976)	Required of mental health professionals a duty to warn that necessitates an evaluation of a patient's potential to become violent toward a specific person
Barefoot v. Estelle (1983)	Expert testimony on dangerousness may not always be correct but it is admissible and the adversarial process should properly evaluate it
Schall v. Martin (1984)	Preventative detention is allowable based on a prediction that the accused poses a serious risk of future criminal conduct
Kansas v. Hendricks (1997) and *Kansas v. Crane* (2002)	Affirmed the constitutionality of sexually violent predator statutes and the use of dangerousness determinations to commit them

risk outside of forensic situations (see Table 5.1 for a summary of these cases).

It is important to examine these cases from a therapeutic jurisprudence perspective. All of these cases support the notion that the law can have a profound impact on the practice of forensic psychology and thereby on the mental health of individuals that come into contact with the legal system. If forensic psychology had responded to these cases with a business-as-usual mentality, individual civil rights and liberty could be at stake along with the mental health of those individuals both incorrectly released because of poor violence risk assessments and those that were institutionalized. The best research available indicated that clinicians were more often wrong than right (Monahan, 1981) and that flipping a coin was more accurate than predictions of violence (Ennis & Litwack, 1974). However, instead of maintaining the status quo, forensic psychologists used these Court decisions to improve the reliability and validity of predictions of dangerousness and improve the therapeutic results.

The Evolution of Risk Assessment

Court cases such as *Barefoot* and *Schall* came at an interesting time for forensic psychology. There was significant pessimism about the ability of forensic psychologists to predict future dangerousness. John Monahan's (1981) famous review of the research concluded that predictions of dangerousness were wrong two out of three times. As a result, there was some surprise when the Supreme Court discounted the state of the scientific literature and continued to encourage this type of expert testimony. Although these court cases certainly were not the only impetus for the continued development of research in predictions of violence (Grisso, 1995), they did provide further encouragement for the heightened interest in the area that occurred in the late 1970s and into the 1980s.

Early History of Risk Assessment

Research on predictions of dangerousness and violence risk assessments have frequently been commented upon in terms of a generational development (e.g., Otto, 1992). The *first generation* of research that occurred during the 1970s largely focused on institutionalized individuals in psychiatric, forensic, and correctional settings awaiting release. The results of this first generation of research, especially the studies comparing mental health professionals' predictions against the outcomes in the community, were so poor that some called for the abolishment of civil commitment (see Monahan, 1981). Monahan (1988) articulated that there were four major shortcomings of this first generation of research. The studies focused on poor predictors of violence, enabled poorly measured and defined violence outcomes, used narrow samples, and were poorly organized (Monahan, 1988). Monahan (1988) further recommended a host of improvements to remedy the problems apparent in this research on violence risk assessment.

Although there is some disagreement about the strides made in the *second generation* of risk assessment research (see Steadman, 1992 for contrary stance), most believed the field made tremendous advances by focusing on short-term predictions and identifying useful predictor variables that were more definitively associated with violence across domains (Otto, 1992; Poythress, 1992). Many studies during the second generation of research focused on short-term predictions, primarily in hospital settings (e.g., McNeil & Binder, 1987, 1991). These foci are in keeping with Monahan's (1988) suggestions as these situations may allow for greater attention to precise data collection and control that would increase the accuracy of forensic psychologists.

Another improvement that set the foundation for the potential *third generation* of risk assessment research was the identification of individual and contextual variables that related to violence. Klassen and O'Connor (1988a, 1988b) conducted some of the most noted research among psychiatric samples. Klassen and O'Connor followed formerly hospitalized patients for upwards of one year post discharge in the community. They identified patients who exhibited violence either via an arrest or readmission to the hospital and those who were non violent. They then identified variables that related to prediction of one of these two groups and were able to classify 88–93% of the patients accurately, though the accuracy decreased when the model was applied to additional samples (Klassen & O'Connor, 1990).

In his review of this second generation of studies, Otto (1992) was cautiously optimistic. He stated that several improvements had been advanced during the last decade such as identifying various outcome or criterion measures beyond arrest records, a moderate base rate of violence for the mentally ill with a previous history of violence, and that mental health professionals have some ability to predict dangerousness. In regard to the third and final conclusion, Otto (1992) stated that "rather than only one in three predictions of long-term dangerousness being accurate, at least one in two short-term predictions of dangerousness behavior are accurate" (p. 130).

A final and very important development was the move from predicting dangerousness to assessing risk of violence (Poythress, 1992). Forensic psychologists historically referred to the process described here as predicting dangerousness, potentially because of the legal tradition involved. However, as the second generation concluded there was encouragement for the use of the phrase, *risk of violence*, for several reasons. Monahan (1992) believed the use of the word dangerousness encouraged dichotomous judgments (the person is dangerous or she is not dangerous) that were in keeping with the dichotomous legal thinking but contrary to the probability of violence (e.g., a 20% probability of future violence) associated with assessing risk from a psychological standpoint. Dichotomous decisions also force potential variables of interest into a single conclusion that ignores the independence of the different factors (Poythress, 1992). We examine risk in different ways to avoid this problem. Also, by focusing on risk of violence, forensic psychologists can clearly identify the variables that present a risk (substance abuse, threats of aggression, violent fantasies) and the variable of interest, the violence (Poythress, 1992).

Assessing risk is not simply a matter of identifying whether someone is going to commit a violent act; there are multiple facets involved in risk assessment (Douglas & Ogloff, 2003). Instead of thinking about risk assessment as only the likelihood of someone becoming violent, it should be viewed as consisting of several different components (Hart, 2005). Hart has suggested there are five different facets to violence risk assessments that include: (1) nature; (2) severity; (3) frequency; (4) imminence; and (5) likelihood. Although many measures designed for risk assessment only take into account likelihood of future violence occurring, it is equally important to consider the other four facets. What is the nature of the potential violence? The forensic psychologist should focus on different predictor variables and potentially have a different outcome if the focus is sexual violence, domestic violence, or general violence. What is the potential severity of the violence? The final decision will be much different if the potential severity is murder compared to a slap on the face. How frequently will the potential violence occur? Someone who is likely to commit repeated violent acts warrants more consideration than someone who is likely to commit a single act of equally severe violence. Finally, what is the imminence of the potential violence? This facet may be especially sensitive to intervention and treatment. If the imminence of the violence is immediate because of unmanaged symptoms of schizophrenia, then the imminence of violence will decrease once the individual is medicated. As a result, modern conceptualizations of risk assessment do not merely focus on the likelihood of the violence but they also focus on additional factors that are equally important.

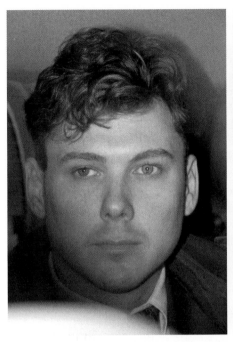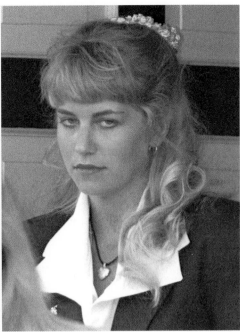

Figure 5.1. Paul Bernardo and his wife, Karla Holmolka, are two of the most notorious serial killers in the history of Canada. His scores on the VRAG are a good illustration of a potential problem with the strict actuarial approach to risk assessment. They are also the subject of Box 5.2 in this chapter. © PA Photos/Canada Press

Structured Professional Judgments

An approach that clearly emerged by the late 1990s was the use of structured risk assessment approaches or **structured professional judgment** (SPJ). SPJ focuses on lists of important risk factors and general guidelines for using those risk factors. Structured approaches to risk assessment are normally based on identification of a list of factors from the relevant scientific literature (Litwack et al., 2006). Structured approaches such as the HCR-20 can be scored similar to an actuarial measure. For example, the HCR-20 is comprised of 20-items focusing on historical, clinical, and risk areas. Each item is scored similar to the PCL-R. If there is no evidence of the presence of an item, it is scored a zero. If there is definitive evidence of a particular item, it is scored a two. A score of one is given if there is some but less than definitive evidence for the presence of a particular item. A list of the HCR-20 items is located in Table 5.2. The difference between a measure like the HCR-20 and an actuarial measure like the COVR is that clinical judgment is encouraged and is necessary in arriving at a final decision for the HCR-20. As a result, an individual like Paul Bernardo may score low on the HCR-20 but the fact that he has killed at least three times and known to have sexually assaulted 75 women would allow the

Box 5.2.   One of Canada's Most Notorious Serial Killers

Paul Bernardo was instantly one of Canada's most famous serial killers and rapists when his heinous crimes came to light in the 1990s. Bernardo and his wife, Karla Holmolka, were accused of killing at least three women and raping at least 75 others. One of those women, was Holmolka's sister whom she killed by overdosing her on a veterinary drug they used to sedate her during the rape. Despite his history of savage rape and murder, Bernardo scores very low on at least one actuarial risk measure, the VRAG. A forensic psychologist scoring Mr. Bernardo on the VRAG likely would arrive at a score of −1 which relates to a 17–31% probability of violence. The highest probably of violence in that range is barely above the 26% level, which Monahan and Silver (2003) identified as the threshold for which judges would identify someone as sufficiently dangerous so that they would not release them. Bernardo fails to score high on the instrument because he lived with his parents through adolescence, was free of any elementary school maladjustment, did not have a history of nonviolent or violent criminal offenses prior to his murder and rape trial, was married, had no previous probation or parole, as well as scoring low on other items. Bernardo is an example of an individual whom most would consider extremely high risk to reoffend but whose score on an actuarial instrument does not match this belief.

Ms. Holmolka was originally thought to be an unwilling accomplice and a victim of Bernardo's sadistic abuse. However, after she agreed to a plea bargain in exchange for her testimony against Bernardo, police found evidence that suggested she was a more willing and active participant than originally thought. Videotape evidence showed that she raped many of the victims herself, other evidence suggests she also may have physically brutalized them, she reportedly studied about battered woman syndrome prior to her trial, and she received media attention for throwing parties with her lesbian lover while in prison. Many experts have suggested that she is an outstanding example of a female psychopath. Despite this evidence and behavior, Holmolka served her complete 12-year sentence and was released in 2005. She has never expressed remorse for her role publicly, was romantically involved with another murderer upon her release, is now married, has given birth to a boy and is living in Quebec.

forensic psychologist to place him at high risk for future violence. As a result, a forensic psychologist could override the decision suggested by the final score on an instrument. However, this practice also increases the chance of bias that actuarial approaches avoid.

The evidence concerning the use of SPJ is also promising. The HCR-20 was originally validated on a sample of civil psychiatric patients but also has been validated on correctional samples (Douglas & Webster, 1999) as well as both inside and outside of North America (Grann, Belfrage, & Tengstrom, 2000). Studies show that the HCR-20 is equal if not superior to actuarial measures in predictive ability (Douglas, Yeomans, & Boer, 2005; Doyle, Dolan, & McGovern, 2002; Grann et al., 2000). There also are structured approaches

Table 5.2. Items from the HCR-20

Historical items	Previous violence
	Young age at first violent incident
	Relationship instability
	Employment problems
	Substance use problems
	Major mental illness
	Psychopathy
	Early maladjustment
	Personality disorder
	Prior supervision failure
Clinical items	Lack of insight
	Negative attitudes
	Active symptoms of major mental illness
	Impulsivity
	Unresponsive to treatment
Risk items	Plans lack feasibility
	Exposure to destabilizers
	Lack of personal support
	Noncompliance with remediation attempts
	Stress

Source: Adapted from Webster, Douglas, Eaves, & Hart (1997)

for assessing domestic violence (Spousal Assault Risk Assessment; SARA) and sexual violence (Sexual Violence Risk-20; SVR-20). Though the evidence is less abundant than for the HCR-20, there is also support for the use of the SARA (Kropp & Hart, 2000) and the SVR-20 (de Vogel, de Ruiter, & van Beek, 2004).

At this time, there is no clear consensus among forensic psychologists as to the best approach for conducting a violence risk assessment. Professionals such as the group in Penetanguishene, Ontario argue for the abandonment of any clinical or structured approaches and a strict use of actuarial measures (Quinsey et al., 2006). Furthermore, they freely admit that their opinion has changed over the years as they have evaluated the developing research (Quinsey, Harris, Rice, & Cormier, 1998). The issue becomes even more complicated as others argue that it is difficult, if not impossible, to separate clinical and actuarial approaches because good clinical practice includes the use of actuarial approaches, though it allows for deviation from the results (Litwack, 2001). The conflict is even more difficult to resolve because of the continued limitations of the current research, some of which are inherent to risk assessment.

Risk and Protective Factors

So far we have talked about some of the general issues relevant to violence risk assessment. However, we have not discussed some of the specific factors relevant to an assessment of future risk. Generally, risk factors for violence can be divided into static risk factors and dynamic risk factors. Static factors are normally fixed and unchanged across time. Dynamic factors tend to be malleable and altered by time or specific forces. One of the previously discussed risk assessment measures, the HCR-20, will serve as a good exemplar for the differences between these two types of risk factors. In addition to risk factors, the importance of protective factors or factors that reduce the risk of violence has been recently examined.

Static Risk Factors

Historical or **static factors** are variables that increase the risk of future violence but are unlikely to change and are often fixed. For example, gender and race are two clearly static factors. A person's gender or race typically does not change over the course of a lifetime. Most static factors are a little less concrete though in terms of their fixed nature. Previous history of violence is generally considered a static risk factor. If an offender or patient has been violent before, that aspect is not going to change. They cannot erase the violent behavior or the legal conviction that may have resulted from it. Of course, if someone has never been violent that can change if she becomes violent. The entire Historical scale of the HCR-20 is comprised of variables that are generally considered to be static. Positive indications of factors like the age at which someone's first violent behavior occurred, history of relationship or employment instability, previous substance abuse, a diagnosis of a mental disorder, psychopathy, early maladjustment, a diagnosis of a personality disorder, or failing during a prior supervision are fixed.

Static factors were some of the first risk factors identified by forensic psychologists as risk factors for future violence and constitute the majority of the risk assessment research (Gardner, Lidz, Mulvey, & Shaw, 1996a). Generally, static factors are more easily identifiable during routine forensic assessments and more objectively defined. Furthermore, static risk factors are most useful in long-term assessments of risk (Hanson & Morton-Bourgon, 2005). However, focusing only on static factors is problematic when assessing risk because like the factors themselves, it treats risk as a fixed entity that does not change over time. Only focusing on static factors suggests that once an individual's risk has been determined, it is never going to change. This view is in conflict with the idea that criminal offenders can be rehabilitated and that psychiatric patients can be successfully treated. More importantly, we know that individual risk does change over time because of individual factors and contextual reasons (Douglas & Skeem, 2005). Nonetheless, most risk assessment measures focus almost exclusively on static variables.

Dynamic Risk Factors

Traditional risk assessment measures that focus on static factors are missing a significant consideration when examining a person's risk, **dynamic factors**. In contrast to static factors, dynamic factors tend to be malleable and responsive to change or intervention. Only more recently have forensic psychologists begun to give consideration to dynamic factors and truly integrate them into their risk assessments (Doren, 2004). The items on the Clinical scale (lack of insight, negative attitudes, psychiatric symptoms, behavioral and affective instability, and unresponsiveness to treatment) and the Risk scale (plans lack feasibility, exposure to destabilizers, lack of social support, noncompliance with medication, and stress) of the HCR-20 provide a list of potential dynamic factors that should be considered in violence risk assessments.

Dynamic risk factors tend to be more difficult to identify and study. However, the job of forensic psychologists is evolving from simply estimating risk one time to ongoing management. As the mental health system becomes more community-based and patients are moved out of institutions, the necessity for interventions to reduce risk or identify the dynamic risk factors associated with risk are even more important (see Douglas & Skeem, 2005). It also tends to be a small percentage of the most seriously disturbed individuals who are committing repeated acts of violence (Gardner, Lidz, Mulvey, & Shaw, 1996b). As a result, the distinction between risk assessment focused on prediction and risk management is important.

Risk assessment and risk management

Another step in the evolution of dangerousness predictions that is dependent on the identification of dynamic risk factors is **risk management** (Monahan & Steadman, 1994). As the focus of risk assessment has shifted from single administrations, suggestive of an ongoing fixed level of risk, to recognition of the need for multiple administrations and risk reduction, the idea of risk management has become important (Heilbrun, 1997). For example, while working on a civil psychiatric unit, I once had a patient who was arrested for a physical confrontation with another homeless man. He arrived at the hospital with active symptoms of schizophrenia and claimed to be a descendant of Pocahontas. Over the course of several weeks and months, his symptoms continually improved and he became more stable. There were several points throughout his treatment that staff were required by law to make a decision regarding his risk and whether he should be released. If we had simply assessed his risk immediately after the assault when his symptoms were active and never changed our evaluation of his potential risk, he would never have been a good candidate for discharge. As his symptoms decreased and he received treatment for a co-occurring substance abuse problem, he became a much better candidate for discharge and eventually was released and did not return to the hospital.

Heilbrun (1997) identified several differences between a prediction oriented model of risk assessment and risk management. First, the central *goal* of risk assessment is to identify whether an individual is likely to become violent at some point in time. The goal of risk management is to reduce the likelihood of aggression. Second, the *nature of the risk factors* in risk assessment is going to be both static and dynamic but in risk management the focus is going to be primarily on dynamic variables that can change in order to reduce violence. Third, the *nature of post assessment control* is also different. In risk assessment, there often is not the ability to supervise individuals continually. Once they are released, they are on their own. In risk management, there must be some ability to monitor and follow people continually in order to assess their progress. Fourth, as our previous discussion already suggests, there is a difference in *the number of administrations*. Risk management necessitates multiple administrations of a violence risk assessment whereas prediction focused risk assessment assumes a single administration. The implications for risk assessments are not that the manner in which risk assessments are conducted should inherently change. Risk management is merely an additional reminder that risk assessment is multifaceted both in terms of the prediction and in terms of the process.

Protective Factors

A final aspect of risk assessment that has been sorely overlooked is the use of protective factors (Rogers, 2000). Most models of risk assessment focus on the factors that are likely to exclusively increase risk without paying attention to the factors that are likely to decrease risk. **Protective factors** are factors that decrease the likelihood of someone committing violence. The suicide prevention literature does a better job at identifying protective factors in assessing suicide risk than the risk assessment literature for violence toward others (Montross, Zisook, & Kasckow, 2005). For example, a person may present significant risk for suicide because of a history of depression, current symptoms of depression, substance abuse problems, and the recent death of a spouse. However, if that same person presents with a very wide and supportive social network of friends and family and has strong religious convictions that strongly discourage suicide; they act as buffers to reduce his likelihood of suicide. The literature on violence toward others is significantly lacking in terms of not only the identification of protective factors but the incorporation of those factors into models of risk assessment. However, recent models for the assessment of risk incorporate so called protective factors (see Doren, 2004).

The definition or conceptualization of protective factors is not always clear. Protective factors are normally factors that interact with risk factors to reduce someone's risk for violence (Rogers, 2000). They offer an explanation for why two people with identical levels of risk may behave differently. Just as risk factors do not guarantee that an individual is going to become violent, protective factors do not guarantee that someone is going to continue being non violent. Moreover, protective factors are not simply the absence of risk factors but themselves reduce, not just fail to increase, the level of risk. That does not mean the absence of a risk factor cannot be a protective factor, just that the absence is not automatically a protective factor. For example, psychopathy is clearly a risk factor for incarcerated criminal offenders in assessing their risk to commit additional violence upon release. However, does the absence of psychopathy reduce one's risk significantly compared to the average offender? The research is largely quiet on that question but we cannot assume that it does simply because of its absence (Rogers, 2000). If you were thinking about going to some warm tropical location for a vacation, would you only think about the reasons not to go (sunburn, spending money, potential hassle of travel)? Or would you consider all the benefits and good things that would come out of it? Considering only the risk factors in making risk assessments is very similar. A forensic psychologist should consider both the risk factors and the protective factors.

Accuracy of Risk Assessment

People often ask, how accurate are we at assessing risk? That question is very difficult to answer with a single percentage or phrase. Rather than being able to definitively state the accuracy of forensic psychologists to assess the risk of violence, it is probably better to identify some of the difficult aspects of violence to assess and some of the situations in which forensic psychologists are good at assessing risk.

Difficulties in Risk Assessment

There are a number of problems that are associated with studying and assessing violence risk. Some of these problems are inherent to assessing violence whereas others continue to be problematic despite Monahan's (1984; 1988) earlier critiques. Several of the difficulties with assessing risk are because of the nature of violence itself. Specifically, it is difficult to obtain accurate follow-up information. Violence is a behavior that is not readily reported or easily identifiable except in extreme cases. Moreover, collection of follow-up data necessitates following individuals who tend to be more transient and less likely to maintain stable and public lifestyles.

A related problem with risk assessment is the measurement of violence. Historically, violence has been measured via formal legal charges and convictions for violent crimes. However, doing so misses the majority of the violence perpetrated because most violence never results in legal charges. Even recent studies focusing on violent recidivism have found different results using two different official criminal databases (Barbaree, 2005: Seto & Barbaree, 1999). The differences between recorded legal charges and actual violence must be only greater. Recent studies have sought to gather additional self-report data from research participants as well as significant others around them (Monahan et al., 2001) in order to improve on this problem. Nonetheless, measuring violence remains problematic.

Our initial discussion of a definition of violence also highlighted one of the problems with studying violence risk assessments. There is a great deal of variability in how violence is defined (Edens & Douglas, 2006). Many people include verbal and physical aggression as violence. Some only define violence in terms of legal convictions. The difficulty comes in comparing results across studies that have divergent definitions of violence and in relying on the convergence of these studies to identify appropriate predictors of violence. If two studies conclude very different things, it may be because their outcome measure, violence, is very different. There may even be different predictors of different severity levels of violence. X list of variables may predict murders and Y lists of variables may predict bar fights.

Another problem is the low base rate of violence (Wollert, 2006). Violence is not a frequently occurring event and therefore it is difficult to study and maintain accurate estimates of risk. If the **base rate** or frequency for violence is 10%, a prediction that no one would become violent would be accurate 90% of the time. Why would a forensic psychologist ever predict violence if the only goal was accuracy? Because there are numerous other goals such as protecting the public and forensic psychologists are not about to start playing the odds. Low base rates further make it difficult for researchers to get a clear indication of the variables that are related to violence. Although there are ways to get around this problem such as using statistical techniques (e.g., Receiver Operating Characteristics) that are less tied to base rates (Mossman, 1994), and lengthy follow-up periods (e.g., 10 years), it is still an issue that continues to hamper violence risk assessment.

When are We Good at Assessing Risk?

There are also a number of situations in which forensic psychologists are good at assessing risk for violence. As the literature has developed, it has become clearer that forensic psychologists are good at assessing risk for short periods of time (Mossman, 1994). It is much easier to assess whether a patient is going to become violent over 48 hours or 14 days than for 48 months or 14 years. A number of factors can change the longer the required follow-up period. An individual may lose his job, get divorced, start drinking alcohol again, or stop taking psychiatric medication. The longer the period of time a single risk assessment administration is to cover, the more room for potential error.

We are also good at assessing risk for people if we have adequate information about their past behavior, especially violent behavior (Elbogen, Huss, Tomkins, & Scalora, 2005). Individuals who are incarcerated for years in a prison or who are chronic patients in a mental hospital are likely to have extensive documentation that provides information about their past behavior. However, in situations where information is lacking or limited, assessment becomes more difficult. For example, assessing risk for a psychotic individual brought into an emergency room without any identification is very difficult if you think back to the historical risk factors identified on the HCR-20 (Table 5.2). How many of those items do you think a forensic psychologist can identify in an unidentified psychotic patient? Forensic psychologists also are good at assessing violence for settings in which they have past data. A forensic psychologist is going to be much more accurate at assessing risk in a person who is released into a community if they have evidence of the general recidivism rate for that specific community.

Finally, it should not be surprising that we are more accurate in situations in which there are high base rates of violence. Generally, the closer the base rate for violence is to 50%, the more accurate risk assessments are likely to be (Quinsey et al., 2006). Assessing violence risk among the general public will always remain low because violence is relatively rare. However, base rates are heightened when risk is assessed in situations in which previously violent individuals are assessed, individuals who exhibit numerous risk factors are identified, or the assessments occur in institutional settings in which violence frequently occurs and is monitored.

Communicating Risk

A final aspect of violence risk assessment that is important to consider is the manner in which risk assessment is communicated to the courts either via testimony or written reports. At first glance, risk communication may seem relatively unimportant because it has largely been ignored until recently (Heilbrun, O'Neil, Strohman, Bowman, & Philipson, 2000). One of the first discussions of the importance of risk communication occurred in Monahan and Steadman's 1996 article. They compared the process of violence risk assessment to weather forecasting, in order to highlight the different ways communication of risk can be important. Weather forecasts often explain the potential for routine weather anomalies in terms of probabilities. For example, there may be a 30% chance of rain for a given day. However, they explain more severe and problematic weather events in terms of categories. For example, there may be a tornado watch (tornado and severe thunderstorms are possible) or a tornado warning (a tornado has been spotted) in instances of severe weather. Monahan and Steadman (1996) also point out that weather forecasters explain the conditions that are likely to lead to the weather event and the steps that should be taken to avoid personal harm in the case of any occurrence. The legal system can only make better informed decisions about risk when mental health professionals communicate that risk in an effective and accurate fashion (Monahan et al., 2002).

There are a variety of ways in which risk can be communicated and the literature is identifying clear preferences among legal actors and mental health practitioners. Research to date has discovered that psychologists prefer to communicate risk in terms of risk management, identification of the relevant risk factors and the potential interventions to reduce the threat of those risk factors. Psychologists also prefer to communicate risk in terms of categorical risk levels (high, medium, and low) over specific probabilities (a 10% chance of becoming violent). Furthermore, Slovic, Monahan, and MacGregor (2000) found that clinicians were more likely to keep a patient hospitalized if the risk were communicated in terms of frequency (20 out of 100) compared to a probability (20%). Monahan et al. (2002) replicated these findings for clinicians working in forensic settings and also found that a more vivid depiction of past victim injuries further increased the likelihood of hospitalization.

These tendencies have direct implications for the preferences of judges and juries. Monahan and Silver (2003) presented judges with information based on the different probability of risk associated with the different risk categories from the MacArthur Risk Assessment Study and asked them to identify the lowest level of risk at which they believed the individual fulfilled the dangerousness criteria for civil commitment. The judges clearly identified the 26% threshold as sufficient for civil commitment. It is interesting that the threshold judges preferred resulted in a 76.8% classification rate. However, this would mean civilly committing a little over one-third of the patients of which over 50% would have been non violent without any civil commitment (Monahan & Silver, 2003). Not only should forensic psychologists thrive to increase the accuracy of their assessments of violence risk but they also should pay attention to the manner in which those determinations are communicated to the court.

Summary

In defining violence for risk assessment purposes, the focus was on violence as a physical behavior that is based on a decision to be violent. This definition is important for psychological as well as legal reasons. There have been a number of developments that have encouraged and shaped violence risk assessment in keeping with the notion of therapeutic jurisprudence. Cases such as *Barefoot v. Estelle* (1983), *Schall v. Martin* (1984), and *Kansas v. Hendricks* (1997) have encouraged the use of violence risk assessments in a variety of settings and, therefore, encouraged improvements in the research and practice of forensic psychology.

The identification of risk assessment in terms of generational changes makes it easier to identify several aspects in the development of risk assessment. Although the first generation of violence prediction was marked by comparisons of flipping a coin and much pessimism, by the third generation of risk assessment significant advancement had taken place. The improvements were characterized by the clear identification of relevant risk factors and the formation of those risk factors into actuarial and structured risk assessment approaches. Even though early research was not supportive of the use of clinical approaches, discussion continues as to the best use of clinical, structured, and actuarial approaches.

As research began to identify risk factors for violence consistently, forensic psychologists further clarified the nature and role of these risk factors.

Recognition of the differences between static and dynamic factors helped acknowledge the limitations of static factors and the need to identify dynamic factors. This recognition occurred as forensic psychologists realized the importance not only of risk assessment but also of risk management. In addition, the importance of protective factors was noted as a relative deficiency compared to static and dynamic risk factors.

Finally, the condition under which a forensic psychologist can make more accurate risk assessment decisions and identification of the impact of risk communication has begun. Violence risk assessments are routinely limited by problems in defining violence, proper follow-up, appropriate and comprehensive measurement, and low base rates for violence. Forensic psychologist are good at assessing risk when they make them for short periods of time, have past data regarding the individual, and there are moderate to high base rates for violence. Use of the relevant research data often culminates in a forensic psychologist needing to communicate her findings to the legal system either via a prepared report or expert testimony. Research is beginning to suggest that the manner in which risk assessment conclusions are communicated can alter the ultimate legal decisions.

Key Terms

actuarial risk assessments	nomothetic
amicus curiae	protective factors
base rate	risk assessment
clinical risk assessments	risk management
dynamic factors	static factors
idiographic	structured professional judgment

Further Readings

Monahan, J., Steadman, H. J., Silver, E., Appelbaum, P. S., Robbins, P. C., Mulvey, E. P., et al. (2001). *Rethinking risk assessment: The MacArthur study of mental disorder and violence.* New York: Oxford University Press.

Quinsey, V. L., Harris, G. T., Rice, M. E., & Cormier, C. A. (2006). *Violent offenders: Appraising and managing risk* (2nd ed.). Washington, DC: American Psychological Association.

Sexual Offenders

There may be no other area of forensic psychology that has undergone as dramatic a change in as short an amount of time as has clinical practice and research involving sexual offenders. The pattern parallels the passage of a host of U.S. legislation and decisions by the U.S. Supreme Court involving sexual offenders (Conroy, 2002). Often when dramatic change occurs in a very short period of time it is accompanied by controversy and this area of forensic practice is no different. Disagreement ranges from simple operational and diagnostic labels involving sexual offenders to the treatment and appropriate use of legal interventions (Conroy, 2002; Marshall, 2006; Quinsey, Harris, Rice, & Cormier, 2006). The majority of the literature and clinical practice has focused on male sexual offenders and as a result this chapter will focus largely on them, with some specific attention to other special populations of sexual offenders such as juveniles, women, and the clergy.

What is a Sexual Offender?

The term sexual offender is likely to bring with it a particularly negative connotation and a myriad of assumptions and stereotypes, both among the general public and forensic psychologists (Geffner, Franey, & Falconer, 2003). Most people think of horrific crimes like those of John Couey. Couey kidnapped 9-year-old Jessica Lunsford from her own bedroom after breaking into her home, sexually assaulted her, and buried her alive. However, there are also sexual offenders similar to the character portrayed by Kevin Bacon in the movie *The Woodsman* (Box 6.1).

As a result, it is important to remember that sexual offenders are a heterogeneous group of offenders from a host of backgrounds and there is significant variety in the type and manner in which they commit their crimes. The term sexual offender is largely a legal term used to label anyone who has committed a sexual offense that is characterized by the use of force or a threat to engage

Box 6.1.   Jessica Lunsford

Jessica Lunsford was an energetic 9-year old-girl, living in Homosassa, FL when she made national headlines after her kidnapping, brutal rape and murder. In February 2005, Jessica was home sleeping when John Couey, who lived in a trailer about 100 yards away, entered her home. He awakened Jessica and ordered her to follow him outside of her home. He took her to his trailer that night where he repeatedly sexually assaulted her before he went to work that morning. Three days after Couey abducted Jessica he bound her limbs, placed her in multiple garbage bags, and buried her alive in a shallow grave where she suffocated. Jessica's body was found three weeks later after intensive searching and a confession by her attacker. John Couey was later convicted of his crimes and sentenced to death. As a result of her attack and death, legislation was proposed in Florida, the Jessica Lunsford Act, and around the country in her name to improve the tracking of released sexual offenders and lengthen prison sentences of convicted sexual offenders.

Though Jessica Lunsford's death was horrific and is often brought up as an example of a typical sexual assault. The circumstances around her death were not the norm for several reasons. For example, most sexual offenders are rapists and not child molesters, though child molesters appear to be becoming inappropriately synonymous with sexual offender and even the more current term sexual predator. Most sexual offenders know their victim and do not break into houses of strangers to commit their crimes or pick up children on their way home from school. Moreover, it is actually rare that a victim of a sexual assault is murdered during or after the attack. Many of the sensationalized media images are not characteristic of all or even most sexual offenders. Kevin Bacon gives a dramatic and realistic portrayal of a sexual offender in the movie *The Woodsman*. This movie depicted many of the difficulties sexual offenders must confront and the ongoing battle many of them experience who do not want to reoffend.

in a sexual act. However, there is also significant variability in the manner in which different jurisdictions define sexual assault (Geffner et al., 2003). Consequently, sexual offenders are a group of offenders that include individuals who molest children, rape adults, expose themselves and view other people engaging in sexual acts. Defining some of these distinct groups is often characterized by a mix of legal terms (e.g., sexual predator) and psychological terms (e.g., pedophile) that overlap but also can conflict in their precise meaning. As a result, it is important to start with a clear description of some of these differences.

The basis for much of the confusion in labels prescribed to sexual offenders is the use of paraphilic diagnoses. A **paraphilia** is a formal mental illness identified in the DSM-IV TR as characterized by "recurrent, intense sexual arousing fantasies, sexual urges or behaviors" that involve: (1) non human objects; (2) suffering or humiliation of oneself or one's partner; or (3) children or other nonconsenting persons (American Psychiatric Association, 2000, p. 566). An individual need not actually perform an illegal act or even a legal behavior to be diagnosed with a paraphilia. The definition of paraphilia includes individuals who simply experience arousing fantasies or sexual urges and therefore an illegal act is not required, though it could be nearly sufficient for a diagnosis. Even engaging in a legal act could cause some to be diagnosed, if the activity is regarded as deviant or necessary for the sexual experience. For example, the television character George Costanza on the show *Seinfeld*, once attempted to watch television and eat a pastrami sandwich while having sex. These activities are all legal but if he was not able to become sexually gratified without them, he could be diagnosed as suffering from a paraphilia. Nonetheless, the current focus on sexual offenders will include only those individuals who have performed an illegal sexual act, which has come to the awareness of the legal authorities.

The confusion is even more complex when the distinction between a specific paraphilia, pedophilia, and child molestation is examined. The term **child molester** is normally used to label anyone who has perpetrated a sexual crime against a child. Although the legal requirements tend to vary across jurisdictions, the general age of sexual consent is between 16 and 18 years of age. A child molester would then be considered any adult who has engaged in a sexual act with anyone under the age of consent. However, a **pedophile** (APA, 2000) is someone involved in sexual activity or experiencing significant distress over sexual urges or fantasies involving a prepubescent individual (normally considered to be age 13 or younger). An individual could be a child molester and not a pedophile or in even more rare circumstances a pedophile and not a child molester. There are some mental health professionals that consider all child molesters pedophiles (Abel, Mittelman, & Becker, 1985) but this stance is not universal (Marshall, 2006). Regardless, there appears to be a clear distinction between the two labels in terms of offending patterns (Marshall, 1998) and though pedophile suggests a mental illness in need of treatment, Marshall (2006) argues that all child molesters need treatment whether they are diagnosed as a pedophile or not. As a result of the potential distinction, the term child molester will be used as the general term and pedophilia as a more narrow term specifying a person with that particular mental illness.

Other definitional issues are less convoluted than the distinction between pedophiles and child molesters. The second major category of sexual offenders, though it represents the greater percentage of sexual offenders (Quinsey et al., 2006), is that of rapists. Unlike child molesters, rapists do not have a parallel diagnosis in DSM-IV TR. Some forensic psychologists tend to use the diagnoses of sexual sadism and **paraphilia NOS** (not otherwise specified) to describe individuals who have perpetrated sexual assaults against adult peers, though the practice seems to occur without any reliability (Doren, 2002; Marshall, 2006; Marshall, Kennedy, Yates, & Serran, 2002). The lack of a single encompassing diagnostic category for rapists probably represents the distinction between the crime of sexual assault and the notion that some sexual offenders may be driven in part by a mental illness to commit their crimes.

Other sexual offenders who less frequently are brought before the legal system tend to be referred to in terms of their paraphilias. **Exhibitionists** display their genitals; **frotteurists** rub themselves against other people, and **voyeurs**, or the more popular term Peeping Toms, view other people nude or engaged in sexual acts. Rather than have hundreds of separate diagnoses listed in DSM, there are other paraphilias such as zoophilia (sexual intercourse with animals) that are classified under the paraphilias NOS category mentioned before. It also should be noted that sexual offenders may suffer from multiple paraphilias or perpetrate on a diverse group of victims.

Assessment of Sexual Offenders

Convicted sexual offenders are typically evaluated in order to assess their future risk or treatment responsiveness. These assessments tend to focus on the phallometric measurement of sexual deviance, the underlying psychological characteristics that are likely to be related to an offender's sexual responsiveness or static and dynamic risk factors that are related to long-term recidivism. These areas also are not mutually exclusive. For example, a sexually deviant response as measured on a phallometric device may be useful to assess treatment effectiveness and long-term risk. However, suspected sexual offenders are, unfortunately, also evaluated to assess whether they committed a particular offense. For example, an individual may reveal a pattern of sexual deviance on a phallometric measure and have it used as evidence that the individual committed a particular crime. This type of clinical practice is similar to the trauma and profile evidence discussed in Chapter 3 and is just as flawed. Experts in the field strongly recommend against the use of sexual offender assessment results to suggest the guilt or innocence of an individual (Marshall, 2006; Quinsey et al., 2006) because it lies outside the scope of practice of forensic psychologists and is not supported by the psychological research. Using this evidence is like saying that because someone eats steak, he is guilty of stealing it from the local grocery store. This same logic has been incorrectly used to suggest that because people exhibit sexual excitement to sexual violence, they are guilty of a particular sexual assault. Appeals court decisions also have found such evidence inadmissible and generally lacking scientific support (*Louisiana v. Hughes*, 2003).

Phallometric Assessment: Penile Plethysmograph (PPG)

Phallometric measures such as the **penile plethysmograph** (see Figure 6.1) are routinely used to determine the sexual preferences of male sexual offenders (Marshall & Fernandez, 2000). A phallometric measure consists of some sort of sexual stimuli, monitoring equipment placed on the individual, and recording equipment. The sexual stimuli are either visual, auditory, or a combination of both. They normally consist of the presentation of audio or video stimuli that are deemed unusual or deviant in some manner along with neutral and sexually appropriate stimuli. Before an individual is exposed to these stimuli, he is

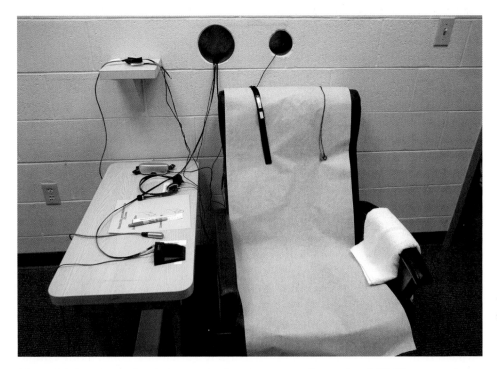

Figure 6.1. A penile plethysmograph prior to use. © eyevine/NY Times

connected to monitoring equipment. The monitoring equipment may consist of devices to measure heart rate, skin conductance (perspiration), and penile engorgement. Any response the individual gives to particular stimuli is then transmitted to the recording equipment and permanently stored either as a hard copy or on a computer.

The underlying notion is that sexual offenders engage in their antisocial sexual behavior because of sexually deviant preferences that are exhibited when they view/hear similar sexual stimuli. The belief is that if an individual exhibits a response to deviant stimuli, they have similar urges and fantasies outside of the testing situation. For example, it would be quite appropriate for a heterosexual male to exhibit an accelerated pulse or penile engorgement if he views sexually suggestive pictures of women and listens to sexually suggestive conversations while doing so. Having a similar response to sexually suggestive pictures of small boys would be considered sexually deviant. Of course, there are legal limitations to the stimuli that can be shown. Nude pictures of children engaged in sexual acts are against the law and are not used. However, pictures of children with accompanying auditory description of a sexual nature could be used.

Phallometric measures are potentially very useful because most sexual offenders are likely to deny attraction to inappropriate situations such as small children or violent sexual activity (Blanchard, Klassen, Dickey, Kuban, & Blak, 2001).

Marshall (2006) even states that almost all reviews of the phallometric literature have come to positive conclusions regarding the use of phallometric measures with child molesters. Studies have found that phallometrics exhibit discriminant validity and are able to differentiate child molesters from non offenders (Chaplin, Rice, & Harris, 1995). Chaplin et al. (1995) compared 15 child molesters who had not been previously tested to 15 non offenders who volunteered from the community. They found very clear discrimination between the two groups, especially in relation to more coercive and brutal stimuli. Several studies also have supported the use of phallometric measures with rapists. In a meta-analysis, Lalumière and Quinsey (1994) examined 17 studies comparing rapists and non rapists on phallometric measures. They concluded that the phallometric literature supported the discrimination between rapists and non rapists across settings, though there was some difference across stimulus materials (Lalumière & Quinsey, 1994).

However, the accuracy of these procedures continues to be challenged (Conroy, 2002). Early beliefs were that phallometric measures would have wide utility among sexual offenders because all sexual offenders had learned or been conditioned to display arousal to their deviant interests. More recent research has suggested that a much more limited range of sexual offenders respond characteristically on these measures (Marshall & Fernandez, 2000). For example, phallometric testing has been largely confined to rapists and child molesters because of the limited utility with other populations. Furthermore, studies have had difficulty discriminating child molesters from other sexual offenders (Hall, Proctor, & Nelson, 1988). Others also argue that the discrimination between child molesters and non offenders is only clear when the child molesters have admitted their sexual deviance and they have multiple victims (Marshall, 2006). This finding is especially problematic in the group of offenders for which a validation of their deviant responses is most useful. Some suggest that phallometric measures are limited to child molesters diagnosed with pedophilia (Marshall & Fernandez, 2000) and research has found some difficulty in discriminating adolescent sexual offenders with female victims, compared to those with male victims, from non offenders (Seto, Lalumière, & Blanchard, 2002). Overall, Looman & Marshall (2005) found that rapists do not exhibit preferences for rape stimuli over consensual sexual stimuli.

Psychological Assessment

In addition to phallometric procedures designed to assess sexual offenders, there are also a number of psychological approaches. Generally, psychological approaches to the assessment of sexual offenders have focused on trying to differentiate sexual offenders from non sexual offenders on the basis of overall psychopathology. However, this research has resulted in limited utility for distinguishing among sexual offenders and other impaired non offender groups (Levin & Stava, 1987; Marshall, 1996). The focus has largely turned away from overall psychopathology toward areas that may serve as the basis for sexual offending. Accordingly, Marshall (2006) identified several target areas of sexual offender assessments, which we will touch upon. These areas can be assessed via clinical interview or other specific psychological measures.

Cognitive distortions, empathy, and sexual fantasies have been three of the most prominent areas of assessment among sexual offenders. Most measures have focused on the **cognitive distortions** of sexual offenders but the majority are fairly face valid and transparent so it is obvious what they are trying to assess. Nonetheless, it is important to assess the thinking errors that are part of the core process for sexual offenders being able to commit their crimes. Sexual offenders frequently create self-serving thought patterns that distort reality and allow them to avoid feeling responsibility for their crimes (Langton & Marshall, 2001). For example, an offender might state that his victim wore suggestive clothing even though the victim was four years old, the victim likes violent sex so the offender was obliging, or that his wife was not receptive to his advances so his daughter was an acceptable alternative. All of these ways of thinking are cognitive distortions that allow or encourage the individual to commit a sexual offense. Several scales have been developed to assess for the presence of cognitive distortions (Abel et al., 1989; Bumby, 1996; Burt, 1980; Nichols & Molinder, 1996) but the research is either unsupportive or is still underdeveloped for them. Even if more research is necessary to develop scales assessing sexual offender specific distortions, cognitive distortions remain an important part of the assessment process via clinical interviews.

Victim empathy also has been a central component of most sexual offender assessments. Although there are general measures of empathy available (Davis, 1983), research suggests that sexual offenders don't have difficulty feeling for other people but that they have a specific inability to feel for their victim (Fernandez & Marshall, 2003; Fernandez, Marshall, Lightbody, & O'Sullivan, 1999), and there are not well validated scales designed specifically for this purpose. As a result, clinical interviews and other collateral record searches may be the best option for forensic psychologists trying to assess the degree of victim empathy exhibited by sexual offender.

The importance of fantasies in the commission of any violence is becoming of interest to forensic psychologists (Grisso, Davis, Vesselinov, Appelbaum, & Monahan, 2000). There are even very crude measures that exist to assess deviant sexual interests via offender's sexual fantasies (Baumgartner, Scalora, & Huss, 2002; Gee, Devilly, & Ward, 2004; O'Donohue, Letourneau, & Dowling, 1997). Baumgartner et al. (2002) used the Wilson Sex Fantasy Inventory to examine differences between child molesters and non sexual offenders. As expected, the child molesters reported more pronounced fantasies across several subscales of the measure and overall reported higher levels of sexual fantasies than did non sexual offenders from a forensic unit. Again, the research supporting the use of measures designed to assess sexual fantasies is preliminary and forensic psychologists are probably much more likely to use clinical interviews to assess sexual fantasies among sexual offenders.

Risk Assessment and Recidivism

Much of the early discussion in the sexual offender literature focused on whether sexual offenders were specialized offenders or sexual offenses were one of many crimes that general offenders committed (Lussier, 2005). This potential distinction is central to the discussion on the recidivism of sexual offenders and the manner clinicians go about assessing risk among individuals who have perpetrated sexual crimes.

Hanson and Bussière (1998) conducted a meta-analysis focusing on the risk factors related to both non sexual offending and sexual offending recidivism. Their study used 87 unpublished and published studies and all studies included information about sexual offenses, non sexual violent offenses and any reoffense. They divided all potential risk factors into either:

- demographic variables (e.g., age, marital status, education);
- general criminality (e.g., any prior offenses, juvenile delinquency);
- sexual criminal history (e.g., prior sex offenses, female child victim);
- sexual deviancy (e.g., phallometric assessment, any deviant sexual preference);
- clinical presentation and treatment history (e.g., failure to complete treatment, empathy for victims);
- developmental history (e.g., negative relationship with mother), and
- psychological maladjustment (e.g., any personality disorder, anger problems).

There were several interesting findings from their study (Hanson & Bussière, 1998). The strongest predictors of sexual recidivism were phallometric responses toward children and deviant sexual preferences. Prior sexual offenses, presence of a stranger victim, early onset of sexual offending, related child victim, antisocial personality disorder, any prior offenses, age, never married, failure to complete treatment, and male victim also were related to sexual recidivism. In addition, there were several factors that were somewhat surprisingly unrelated to sexual recidivism given the focus of assessment and treatment among sexual offenders. Empathy for victims, denial of a sexual offense, low motivation for treatment, and being sexually abused as a child were all unrelated to sexual recidivism. Overall, only 13.4% of 23,393 sexual offenders recidivated within the average 4–5 year follow-up. However, Hanson and Bussière (1998) believe this figure is an underestimate of the percentage who actually committed additional sex offenses because of undetected offenses.

Similar factors predicted non sexual violence and general recidivism. Recidivists tended to be young, single and of a minority race. They also engaged in a variety of criminal behavior as a juvenile and as an adult. Recidivists of both types of crimes also were more likely to exhibit antisocial personality disorder or psychopathic characteristics. The number of prior sexual offenses and sexual deviancy were unrelated to non sexual violent recidivism. Rapists were more likely to recidivate with non sexual violent crimes than child molesters, thereby suggesting a greater likelihood of specialization for child molesters and more general criminal behavior for rapists. In general sexual offenders also were more likely to reoffend with a non sexual offense than a sexual offense.

Hanson and Morton-Bourgon (2005) updated the earlier meta-analysis and again found that sexual offenders were less likely to recidivate for a sexual offense (13.7%) than a non sexual offense (36.2%). Their findings also suggest factors that are related to repeat sexual offending may not be the same as those factors that are related to initiating sexual offenses. Although adverse family backgrounds and internalization of psychological distress are common in sexual offenders, they did not relate to sexual recidivism. The repeat sexual offender appears similar to the repeat non sexual offender in that he leads an unstable and antisocial lifestyle but different in the sense that he tends to focus on sexually deviant thoughts during periods of stress (Hanson & Harris, 2000).

In general, recidivism rates for sexual offenders vary between studies and with the length of follow-up time. Most of the research suggests that recidivism rates for sexual offenders are similar to Hanson and colleagues' findings. They concluded that 10–15% of sexual offenders recidivate after 5 years. About 20% of sexual offenders recidivate after 10 years and 30–40% after 20 years (Hanson, Morton, & Harris, 2003). However, these figures are probably underestimates because they rely on legal charges and convictions. Hanson et al. (2003) state that it is reasonable to believe that these recidivism rates are underestimates by 10–15%. Nevertheless, it should be equally clear that not all sexual offenders reoffend and that evidence suggests that a minority of sexual offenders recidivate, especially within a decade after release.

In addition to the findings as they relate to sexual offenders generally, special care should also be given to differentiating among rapists and child molesters and even between specific types of child molesters. In general, **intrafamilial child molesters** are less likely to recidivate than rapists or **extrafamilial child molesters** (Hanson & Bussière, 1998). However, age of the offender was a significant intervening variable for child molesters (Hanson, 2002). This finding is in keeping with our knowledge of the average age between different types of sexual offenders. Rapists tend to be younger than child molesters and their risk for recidivism decreases as they age (Hanson, 2002). Extrafamilial child molesters exhibit minimal decline in risk until after age 50, with the highest risk between age 25 and 35 years old. Intrafamilial child molesters appear to be at greatest risk at substantially younger ages though their overall recidivism rate (8%) is lower than rapists (19%) and extrafamilial child molesters (17%) (Hanson, 2002). Intrafamilial molesters who offend against male victims are at lower risk than intrafamilial child molesters who victimize girls (Hanson et al., 2003).

Similar to the literature on general risk assessment, research is increasingly focusing on dynamic variables among sexual offenders. Given the increased focus on the treatment and continued confinement of sexual offenders until treatment progress is demonstrated, it could be argued that dynamic factors are especially important in assessing risk in sexual offenders (Doren, 2002). Hanson and Harris

(2000) collected information on dynamic risk factors for over 400 sexual offenders from file reviews and interviews with their community supervision officers. Sexual offenders who recidivated within 5 years, generally lacked social support, exhibited attitudes tolerant of sexual assault, led antisocial lifestyles, were uncooperative with supervision, and exhibited poor self-management compared to a similar number of sexual offenders who did not recidivate. The recidivists also exhibited elevated levels of anger and distress immediately prior to recidivism. In their previously described meta-analysis, Hanson and Morton-Bourgon (2005) identified similar results. Sexual preoccupations, impulsivity, antisocial attitudes, and intimacy deficits all exhibited small relationships with sexual recidivism. However, psychological distress was not related to recidivism. This finding could be similar to Hanson and Harris' (2000) finding that overall mood did not differ between recidivists and non recidivists in their sample. It may be that psychological distress does not predict recidivism in general but is an immediate precursor in sexual offenders who recidivate.

Risk Assessment Instruments for Sexual Offenders

Similar to the debate regarding general risk assessment, there continues to be debate among forensic psychologists as to the role of clinical, structured, and actuarial approaches. Some of the same arguments against actuarial tools to assess sexual violence have been raised (Grubin, 1999; Sjösted & Grann, 2002) as well as the counter arguments against use of clinical and structured approaches (Hanson et al., 2003; Quinsey et al., 2006). Nonetheless, the proliferation of instruments (structured or actuarial) to assess sexual violence has been dramatic. Over the past decade or so there are easily a dozen different instruments identifiable in the literature and almost half that many have been the focus of considerable research. As a result, the focus of the current discussion will not be on rehashing some of the previous arguments regarding clinical versus actuarial assessment but on examining some of the instruments currently in widespread use to assess sexual violence. Though there is an ever increasing abundance of sexual violence risk assessment instruments (e.g., Minnesota Sex Offender Screening Tool-Revised, Rapid Risk Assessment for Sexual Offence Recidivism, Risk Matrix 2000, Sex Offender Need Assessment Ruling, Structured Anchored Clinical Judgment), our discussion will focus on the Sexual Violence Risk-20 (SVR-20), Sexual Violence Risk Appraisal Guide (SORAG), and the Static-99 (see Table 6.1 for the items on each measure).

The SVR-20 is the only structured approach to the assessment of sexual violence among the major risk assessment measures. The SVR-20 is a 20-item measure scored on a 0–2 points scale similar to the HCR-20 and PCL-R (Boer, Hart, Kropp, & Webster, 1997). In addition, when an item is coded as being present the assessor should indicate whether there has been a recent change (as defined by occurring in the past year) in that item to make it more useful in risk management decisions. Although the SVR-20 is scored, the final point total does not correspond to a probability of risk (e.g., 80% of reoffending in

treatment dropouts. When the studies comparing completers and dropouts were removed from the meta-analysis, there were not treatment differences (Harris, Rice, & Quinsey, 1998). Although Hanson et al. (2002) found group differences, it is not completely clear that the group differences were the result of treatment as opposed to differences in the research designs of the included studies. Lalumière et al. (2005) have further criticized this meta-analysis because the removal of studies with random assignment of participants resulted in no differences between the sexual offenders who received treatment and the offenders who did not receive treatment. Lalumière et al. ultimately conclude that there are probably too few well-controlled studies for a meta-analysis to offer definitive conclusions on the effectiveness of sexual offender treatment programs. Though there may not be a clear consensus about the effectiveness of treatment for sexual offenders, the literature is not as pessimistic as Furby et al. (1989) were many years ago.

Components of Potentially Successful Programs

In addition to trying to assess the effectiveness of sexual offender treatment, there also is some evidence for the components that make up a well-designed treatment program. Early attempts at sexual offender treatment were often behaviorally focused but soon treatment providers encouraged awareness of the cognitive components of sexual offending (Abel, Blanchard, & Becker, 1978) and an awareness of the relapse prevention model (Pithers, Marques, Gibat, & Marlatt, 1983). Cognitive and cognitive-behavioral treatments focus on the relationship between distorted thinking patterns and maladaptive behaviors. Cognitive-behavioral components focus on offender minimization, denial, and victim harm. The goal is to reduce the offender's denial and minimization of the offense and to come to terms with the harm they have inflicted on the victim (Marshall, 1996). Denial and minimization often function as a way to protect the offender from realizing the true consequences of his behavior and many programs believe these issues must be confronted for the sexual offender to effectively participate in treatment (Marshall, 1996). The cognitive-behavioral approach also addresses the attitudes and beliefs about women and children that are likely to result in sexual offense behaviors or sexually deviant interests that lead to the inappropriate behavior. Attitudes that completely sexualize women and view children as the sexual equivalent to adult peers are issues that are frequently addressed.

There are often a variety of deficits underlying the behavior of the sexual offender. For example, low self-esteem and sexual inadequacy often lead to deviant sexual interests (Marshall, 2006). By addressing the lack of self-esteem and sexual inadequacy, the deviant sexual interests will be diminished. Programs also target inadequate interpersonal skills and social functioning. Studies have found that programs that address issues such as anger control, assertiveness training, communication skills, and relationship skills are effective (McGrath, Cumming, Livingston, & Hoke, 2003). Another component often addressed in sexual offender treatment programs is substance abuse. Research suggests that substance abuse and dependence often accompany sexually inappropriate behavior and that it may act as a way to diminish the natural and cultural inhibitions against perpetrating sexually inappropriate behavior (Marques & Nelson, 1989).

Relapse prevention focuses on identification of the series of events that led to sexual offending behavior in the past and ways to replace the thoughts and behaviors that led to inappropriate sexual behavior. This approach was borrowed from the substance abuse field. Just as an alcoholic would avoid bars, a child molester would identify locations where children would be present (e.g., circus, zoo, playgrounds) and similarly avoid them. In addition, child molesters need to realize that certain stressful events such as the loss of a job or argument with a partner might lead to sexual acting out and that they should identify appropriate coping responses when they are faced with these situations. This process is meant to alert the offender when he potentially poses an increased risk to reoffend so he can address the circumstances directly in order to avoid the events that lead to the inappropriate sexual behavior. In addition to the relapse prevention approach used in their program, Marques et al. (2005) recommended several improvements for their original treatment program. They recommended individually tailored treatment with regard to intensity and content, continued monitoring of treatment progress to ensure participants were truly getting the objectives of the program, and an individualized aftercare program.

A final component that can be successful in the treatment of sexual offenders is a pharmacological approach (Hall, 1995). Pharmacological approaches consist of administering drugs that reduce sexual arousal (Lalumière et al., 2005). These drugs usually reduce testosterone thereby reducing the likelihood of physical arousal, sexual fantasies and sexual interest in general (Bradford, 1985). In addition, medications commonly used to treat depression and anxiety, selective serotonin reuptake inhibitors (SSRIs), have been used because they commonly produce side effects related to reduced sexual interest. Pharmacological approaches may hold some promise but definitive conclusions regarding their effectiveness are not possible at this time (Miner & Coleman, 2001). One significant issue with the drugs that seek to reduce sexual interest is that many sexual offenses are not about the offender obtaining sex but are related to a host of other personal issues such as power and control over victims or their own inadequacies.

Special Groups of Sexual Offenders

The discussion has focused on adult male sexual offenders because the overwhelming majority of sexual assaults are perpetrated by adult men. However, there are several special groups of sexual offenders that are receiving increased attention, whether from the media or the psychological literature. Each of these groups has their unique characteristics and challenges.

Juvenile Sexual Offenders

During 2001, over 12,000 juveniles were arrested for sexual assault and other sexual crimes in the United States (U.S. Department of Justice, 2002). The problem of juvenile sexual violence is not limited to the United States as 23% of individuals charged or convicted of sexual offenses in the United Kingdom are between 10 and 21 years old (Home Office, 1998). Despite the fact that juvenile sexual offenders appear to represent almost one quarter of all sexual offenders and that many adult offenders begin their sexual offenses as juveniles (Abel, Osborn, & Twigg, 1993), there has been much less attention given to juvenile sexual offenders than adult offenders. Nonetheless, there has been an increase in the attention paid to juvenile sexual offenders (Zgourides, Monto, & Harris, 1997). Moreover, juvenile offenders appear to present unique challenges for forensic psychologists.

There are many unique challenges to assessing risk among juvenile sexual offenders. Our prior discussion clearly suggested there is a significant emphasis on static risk factors in risk assessment and juvenile offenders obviously have had less time to engage in these risk factors or even reach the normal developmental milestones at which they would be possible (e.g., marriage). As a result, there may be less information on which to base these decisions for juvenile sexual offenders. There is some evidence that the base rate of sexual violence for juveniles may be low in comparison to that of adult sexual offenders (Prentky, Harris, Frizell, & Righthand, 2000), which would make the risk assessment even more difficult. However, the base rate for general recidivism for juvenile sexual offenders is much higher (Witt, Bosley, & Hiscox, 2002). Although there are a number of actuarial and structured instruments available for use with adult offenders and a significant amount of research supporting their use, the research on the reliability and validity for juvenile risk assessment measures is limited (e.g., Righthand et al., 2005). There also is disagreement about the application of adult risk factors to juvenile sexual offenders in the absence of well-established juvenile risk assessment measures (Witt et al., 2002). However, this practice is changing with the identification of some actuarial approaches to sexual violence risk assessment in juveniles.

Although juvenile sexual offending has been identified as a serious problem, the research has almost focused entirely on risk factors. Furthermore, though treatment programs have increased over the past 20 years, there has been little research evaluating the effectiveness of these treatment programs (Ertl & McNamara, 1997). Reviews of the literature suggest that juvenile treatment programs appear to focus on similar components to their adult counterparts (e.g., deviant sexual arousal, social skills, anger control, substance abuse, relapse prevention) and are largely cognitive-behavioral (Ertl & McNamara, 1997). Despite the limited information on treatment success, there does appear to be reason for optimism (Fanniff & Becker, 2006).

Female Sexual Offenders

The prevailing view has been that sexual offending was largely a product of male sexual behavior but current events are increasingly confronting our society with the female sexual offender. Women with names such as Mary Kay Letourneau and Debra Lafave have been appearing in newspaper headlines with increasing regularity because of their sexual crimes (Box 6.2). Although these sensational images have been prevalent in the media, there is relatively little research on female sexual offenders.

Although men continue to perpetrate sexual crimes at a much higher rate than women, the prevalence of sexual crimes perpetrated by women is unknown with estimates ranging from 20 to 300 to one (Christiansen & Thyer, 2002) with about 2% to 5% of all convicted sexual offenders being women (U.S. Department of Justice, 1999). In addition, these data are probably underreports because of difficulty viewing women as sexual offenders. Studies indicate that female sexual perpetrators may be more prevalent among adolescents, around 5% to 7% (Camp & Thyer, 1994; U.S. Department of Justice, 2002). Furthermore, research suggests that female sexual offenders resemble male sexual

---

Box 6.2.   The Case of Mary Kay Letourneau

Headlines about the sexual assault of a child at the hands of an adult offender have unfortunately become commonplace. However, these reports typically involve male perpetrators but women are more frequently perpetrating these crimes. For example, Debra Lafave was a 24 year-old, reading teacher in Florida who was married and appeared to be healthy and attractive before she was charged and convicted of illegal sexual behavior with a minor. In 1997, Mary Kay Letourneau became arguably the first case to make national and international news as a female sexual offender. Mrs. Letourneau came to national prominence after she was charged with statutory rape for engaging in an ongoing sexual relationship with her then 13 year-old pupil, Vili Fualaau. Mrs. Letourneau had taught Fualaau both as a second grade student and then as a sixth grade student. She later pled guilty and was sentences to 89 months in prison. Two months prior to

her guilty plea, Letourneau gave birth to Fualaau's daughter.

Not only was Mary Kay Letourneau's case unusual because of her gender but also because of the ongoing nature of her relationship with Vili Fualaau. Letourneau was released from jail after only serving six months of a suspended sentence under the conditions that she attend treatment and have no additional contact with Fualaau. However, she was found in a car with Fualaau with evidence that they were going to leave the country. She was returned to prison to serve out the remaining years of her prison sentence. Letourneau gave birth to the couple's second daughter with Fualaau about nine months after she had been originally released. She was ultimately released in 2004 after completing her sentence and then married Fualaau, who was 21 years of age. Since then the couple has lived together as husband and wife and she now goes by the name Mary Kay Fualaau.

offenders in a number of ways including family backgrounds, peer relationships, sexual compulsivity, anger, and low self-esteem (Christiansen & Thyer, 2002). Contrary to many expectations, female sexual offenders may be more feminine than female non sexual offenders (Pothast & Allen, 1994) and many female sexual offenders find the crimes sexually arousing, it is not simply a matter of the need for power and control (Matthews, Matthews, & Speltz, 1991). Female sexual offenders also use a host of techniques ranging from violence (beating and burning) and threats of violence to emotional abuse when attempting to silence their victims (Saradjian, 1996; Wolfers, 1993).

It also appears the stereotypical teacher–student relationship portrayed in many media images is not the norm for female sexual offenders and they are a much more diverse group than previously believed. Christiansen and Thyer (2002) identified several different types of female sexual offenders. The *teacher/lover* offenders tend to seek out idealized relationships with young boys. *Intergenerationally predisposed* offenders are women from families with histories of several generations of sexual abuse. The *male-coerced* offender is coerced into sexual offenses by their partner and is often passive and powerless in interpersonal relationships. The *non-relative caregiver/babysitter* offender perpetrates her sexual offenses as a formal babysitter or more informally watching someone's children on occasion. Finally, the *incestuous type* of offender is largely composed of women who perpetrate sexual violence against their children but also include other family relationships such as aunts and sisters. In potentially the largest single study involving female sexual offenders, Ferguson and Meehan (2005) examined 279 convicted female sexual offenders in Florida. They found that the overwhelming number of women used force (86.1% with 17.3% using mutilation or disfigurement), 97.3% were the primary perpetrators, 67.7% of the victims were between 12 and 16 years of age, and they gradually became more violent with age.

Clergy as Sexual Offenders

A group of sexual offenders that has received even more attention and public scrutiny than women who sexually offend are clergy who have sexually offended. Although there have been incidents of clergy from a variety of religious backgrounds sexually molesting children, the crisis was especially acute in the United States for Roman Catholic priests (Plante, 2003). John Geoghan was a defrocked Roman Catholic priest who was a convicted child molester with over 100 accusations of molestation against him. While he was serving his 10 year prison sentence, Geoghan was strangled to death by another inmate in 2004. Although John Geoghan is often used as an iconic example of sexually offending clergy who assault alter boys and school age children, little is actually known about clergy who sexually offend (Songy, 2003). The absence of research probably should not be surprising given the social conventions that are especially strong when it comes to clergy and sexually offending (Sapp, 2005) and the potential unease between mental health professionals and the Catholic Church.

There are a number of myths surrounding sexual abuse by clergy that research has addressed. Several hypotheses have been raised for clerical sexual offenders such as sexual celibacy and a greater prevalence of sexual victimization among perpetrators. However, the limited research available has contradicted these potential reasons (Langevin, Curnoe, & Bain, 2000). Despite the view that child molesters are rampant in the Catholic Church, the best available evidence suggest that only between 2% and 4% of Catholic priests are child molesters (John Jay Report, 2004; see Plante, 2003 for a review). Many believe that the offending clergy have sexual offense histories similar to John Geoghan but research suggests that the overwhelming majority of clergy have fewer than 10 victims each (John Jay Report, 2004; Rossetti, 2002). Most of the victims in these instances are pubescent boys, not young children or girls (Plante, 2003). Although specific interventions or assessment strategies have not been empirically established for use with clergy (Songy, 2003), the available research suggests reduced recidivism rates comparable to non clergy (Rossetti, 2002).

One of the most comprehensive studies ever conducted, focused on sexual offending clergy in the Roman Catholic Church (John Jay Report, 2004). Researchers at John Jay College worked with the Roman Catholic Church to get a comprehensive picture of the nature of the problem in the United States. The study surveyed each diocese across the United States asking for every allegation, not criminal conviction or even credible allegation but every allegation of sexual abuse from 1950 to 2002. This study was unique in that a small sample was not studied but the entire population of Catholic Priests for over half a century was used. Results supported but also contrasted with some earlier findings. Most allegations were against parish priests who were age 25 to 39 at the time of the first allegation. About one-third of the priests suffered from substance abuse problem and only 6.8% reported being sexually abused themselves. Contrast this figure with earlier reviews that suggested a majority of offending priests were sexually abused (Plante, 2003). About 3% of the accused priests had 10 or more allegations against them and 40% of the incidents are alleged to have occurred in a home or parish residence. Even more surprising was that police investigated only 15% of these allegations, only 5% of the clergy were charged and only 2% were convicted (John Jay Report, 2004).

Sexual Offender Legislation

Beginning in the 1990s there was an explosion of legislation targeting all sexual offenders. These laws have largely been aimed at detaining rather than rehabilitating sexual offenders and have frequently been preceded by public outcry after well-publicized sexual crimes (Garlund, 2005). Although the purpose of these laws is to increase public safety, the proliferation of sexual offender legislation offers a unique opportunity to examine the potential therapeutic and anti-therapeutic impact on the offenders themselves and the impact on the practice of forensic psychology. There have been three primary types of laws passed in the past decade: registration and notification laws, residency laws, and sexual predator laws.

Registration and Notification Laws

Sexual offenders are now required to register with local law enforcement in all 50 states of the United States (Schopp, Pearce, & Scalora, 1998). This change in the law is directly attributable to the kidnapping and disappearance of a boy, Jacob Wetterling, in Minnesota in 1989. As Jacob was returning home with his brother and a friend, the children were approached by an armed man that commanded the other two boys to run away after which he kidnapped Jacob. The crime remains unsolved and Jacob continues missing. As a result, the United States Congress passed the 1994 Jacob Wetterling Act which encouraged states to create registration requirements for sexually violent offenses. Another crime against a child led to the formation of sexual offender notification laws in the United States. Megan Kanka disappeared from her home in New Jersey in 1994. A neighbor who had been convicted of two prior sexual offenses later confessed to the brutal kidnapping, rape, and murder of Megan. The United States passed the federal Megan's Law in 1996 and it required the public notification of sexual offenders. Though registration and notification laws are often separate, they frequently work in conjunction with one another across the United States. Registration laws require individuals to contact local law enforcement agents if they have been convicted of sexual crimes while community notification provisions allow the government to make certain information available to the public. Public notification occurs in a variety of ways including posting names and faces of offenders on websites and notifying local schools, daycares, and nursing homes if a sexual offender moves nearby. The criteria for registration and subsequent notification varies across states with 31 states deciding it on an individual basis considering the risk of recidivism and the other 19 states ignoring the relevance of risk (Scott & Gerbasi, 2003). So far, the United States Supreme Court has upheld the constitutionality of these laws based on the challenges before them (*Connecticut Department of Public Safety v. Doe*, 2003). The question remains though, are these laws therapeutic or anti-therapeutic?

There have been numerous objections to these laws that originally were proposed and passed with the intent to protect society. These laws fail to take into account the difficulty a sexual offender may face integrating back into society and the additional burden these procedures place on him that may increase the risk for reoffense (Edwards & Hensely, 2003). The sexual offender typically copes with additional stress by retreating into his sexually deviant thoughts and behaviors. Those laws that are based on identifying a subset of sexual offenders for inclusion as sexual offenders who must register or are subject to notification, often rely on risk assessment procedures that are untested or have limited support. Many states have created their own risk assessment measures with unknown reliability or validity in the peer reviewed psychological literature. Concerns also have been raised about the potential impact on the family and children of known sexual offenders. Children of registered sexual offenders may now be exposed to emotional abuse from peers, victims may now be subject to unwanted attention because of the public notification, and some states have seen a decrease in the reporting of incest offenses and juvenile sexual offenses because families are unwilling to face the possibility of negative publicity for their family (Edwards & Hensely, 2003; Freeman-Longo, 1996; Winick, 1998). There is even concern that public notification laws will simply shift the burden to areas where the sexual offender is unknown, increase the likelihood of more stranger-based crimes, and decrease the likelihood of self-reports and treatment seeking behavior of institutionalized inmates (Edwards & Hensely, 2003). Nonetheless, sexual offenders have reported that despite the potential embarrassment over notification laws, they are likely to increase their incentives to avoid reoffense and increase their commitment to treatment (Elbogen, Patry, & Scalora, 2003). However, an evaluation of Washington's community notification law found that it had little impact on reducing sexual or general recidivism but did speed up the time between an offense and an arrest of a suspect (Schram & Milloy, 1995).

Residency Laws

Residency laws are separate from registration and notification laws but their aims are similar: to keep potentially dangerous individuals away from potential victims. Residency laws vary tremendously but generally require that sexual offenders live anywhere from 500 ft to a quarter of a mile away from locations such as bus stops, schools, parks and daycares (Levenson & Cotter, 2005). Concerns over the potential anti-therapeutic effects of residency laws arise for several reasons. The evidence clearly supports the idea that 90% of sexual assaults occur against known victims, not random strangers at local playgrounds and schools. Research has found that child molesters who reoffend tend to be scattered across a community, not overly represented near these target areas (Colorado Department of Public Safety, 2004) and sexual offenders may be more likely to travel outside of their neighborhood for victims (Minnesota Department of Corrections, 2003). However, studies remain only preliminary and are far from conclusive. Legislation also may make it impossible or nearly impossible for sexual offenders to find housing and therefore increases the odds of them clustering in already high-crime areas or increase the stressors that lead to reoffense (Levenson & Cotter, 2005). Sexual offenders have reported that housing restrictions are likely to increase their isolation, increase financial hardships, and decrease their overall stability (Levenson & Cotter, 2005).

Sexually Violent Predator Laws

Sexually violent predator (SVP) laws tend to be the most controversial and the most complex of the recent sexual offender legislation. At the last count, at least 16 states and the District of Columbia had passed SVP laws that provided for the identification and civil commitment of identified sexual offenders (Fitch, 2003; Kendall & Cheung, 2004). SVP laws tend to be more limited in scope and only seek to identify those sexual offenders who are the most dangerous. Despite potential concerns that the majority of sexual offenders would be identified as SVPs, evidence suggests under 10%, if not under 5%, of sexual offenders across the relevant states have been identified as SVPs (Kendall & Cheung, 2004). Though these laws vary across jurisdictions, SVP laws focus on convicted sexual offenders and provide for the civil commitment of those individuals normally identified as mentally ill and likely to commit a future sexual offense if released. As a result, these laws are similar to civil commitment, which we will discuss in Chapter 9. However, they especially target convicted sexual offenders, not any person who may be mentally ill and dangerous. Normally, sexual offenders who are potential SVPs are identified by local law enforcement or district attorneys and must receive an SVP hearing. During the hearing, both sides present evidence before a judge or jury that the individual should or should not be designated a **sexual predator** or sexually violent predator. If found to be a sexual predator or sexually violent predator, the person is institutionalized after he has served his criminal sentence and receives treatment until he is no longer deemed to be a sexual predator (Fitch, 2003). Texas is the lone exception where SVPs are committed as outpatients and in Virginia and Arizona SVPs can be committed as outpatients or continue their institutionalization as inpatients in a mental health facility (La Fond, 2003). Therefore the term sexual predator indicates a sexual offender at heightened risk to reoffend after release from prison, not anyone who has committed a sexual offense.

SVP laws have been criticized for a variety of reasons. First, SVP laws provide for the continued incarceration of an individual who has already served his sentence for a crime. In essence, it has been argued that they are tried twice for the same crime. There is a prohibition against such practices, *double jeopardy*, in the Constitution of the United States (see Mercado, Schopp, & Bornstein, 2005). Specifically, these laws are based on the likelihood of future crimes, not because they have committed a crime and gone unpunished for it. It could be argued that SVP laws are similar to the movie, *Minority Report* staring Tom Cruise, in which he serves as a futuristic police officer who arrests people who are going to murder someone, as predicted by the premonitions of three special psychic individuals. In no other instance, are convicted offenders institutionalized because they are likely to commit a particular crime instead of the commission of an actual crime. Third, others have argued that these laws amount to Ex Post Facto laws or laws passed after the person has been convicted and are therefore unconstitutional (see Mercado et al., 2005). Despite these concerns, the United States Supreme Court has rejected these as constitutional challenges and found SVP laws to be legally appropriate (*Kansas v. Crane*, 2002; *Kansas v. Hendricks*, 1997).

Additional concerns relate to the assumptions about forensic psychology that are inherent in these laws. The law assumes that forensic psychologists can accurately predict the likelihood of future sexual offending (See Box 6.3 for legislation that may remove psychologists from conducting risk assessments on sexual offenders) with a sufficient degree of certainty that warrants continued institutionalization, potentially indefinitely (see Levenson, 2004). In Minnesota and Washington, where the first SVP laws were passed, very few individuals (less than 4%) identified as SVPs have been released and allowed back in the community (as cited in Fitch, 2003). As a result, states have experienced a number of housing problems and increased costs as their number of institutionalized sexual predators has grown (Fitch, 2003). The state of Washington built an entirely new facility simply for the purpose of housing these individuals (La Fond, 2003). California budgeted 47 million dollars for their SVP program in its second year of existence (as cited in Fitch, 2003). Many critics also point to the debate about the effectiveness of treatment for sexual offenders and question whether legal statutes can rely on the future release of someone because of a reduction in risk due to treatment when it is not clear that treatment is even

Box 6.3.   Could Forensic Psychologists Be Doing Fewer Risk Assessments on Sex Offenders?

As we have discussed in this chapter and in Chapter 5, the use of psychological risk assessment has expanded exponentially in the past 20 years. There is no other area in which it has expanded more than with sexual offenders. The host of new sexual offender legislation has necessitated that evaluations determine the future risk that these offenders pose to the public before they are released, have to register as a sexual offender, or are civilly committed as a sexually violent predator. We have additionally discussed the problems that forensic psychologists have in assessing the risk accurately of anyone, much less sexual offenders. The Adam Walsh Child Protection and Safety Act of 2006 established a national sexual offender registry that incorporated the use of DNA evidence and the tracking of convicted sexual offenders via a global positioning system, increased mandatory minimum sentences and penalties for sex related crimes, increased funding to local law enforcement for tracking these offenders, and created a national registry to prevent

children from being adopted by sexual offenders.

In order to classify sexual offenders for purposes of the law, a three tiered classification system was proposed. However, instead of the court determining the risk level and accompanying tier with the assistance of a risk assessment conducted by a forensic psychologist, all risk levels are assigned based strictly on previous offense history with sexual offenders who have been convicted of more severe crimes to Tier III. Offenders who commit less severe crimes are assigned to Tier II and all other convicted sexual offenders are assigned to Tier I. Such a system may eliminate the need for psychological risk assessments and the accompanying problems but it also treats all offenders who have been convicted of certain crimes the same, no matter their individual differences. It remains to be seen whether such a classification system will be universally adopted or if it is better than the traditional risk assessments performed by forensic psychologists.

effective (Janus, 2000). Despite these criticisms and potential anti-therapeutic consequences, SVP laws continue to be passed and are necessitating an ever increasing presence for forensic psychologists.

Summary

Sexual offenders are generally defined by the crimes they commit but also are a very diverse group and the label, sexual offender, is not always clearly descriptive. In addition to being defined by the crimes they commit, there are also a number of mental illnesses that are characterized by sexual behavior. Paraphilia is the general term used to describe individuals who suffer from these sexual disorders but not all sexual offenders suffer from a paraphilia.

Assessment of sexual offenders often serves a different purpose than assessment of most mental health clients. Assessment of sexual offenders does not serve to identify them as a sexual offender but instead occurs to assess treatment related changes. Sexual offenders are assessed using phallometric measures and a host of psychological approaches focused on domains believed to be integral to the development and perpetration of sexual offenses. Phallometric measures are identified by some as integral for assessing sexual offenders and paraphilias but remain somewhat controversial. There are several psychological measures used for assessing psychological aspects of offending, with no single approach or measure identified as sufficient, but forensic psychologists are probably more likely to assess these different dimensions using clinical interviews or other collateral records.

A great deal of information has been collected about the sexual and non sexual recidivism of sexual offenders. It is important to not only focus on sexual recidivism but also on non sexual recidivism because of the tendency for sexually related crimes to appear as non sexual convictions. Though the risk factors for sexual violence have often been treated as applying to all sexual offenders, there also appears to be differences between child molesters and rapists in their sexual offense patterns. The identified risk factors have been incorporated into a number of risk assessment measures that have demonstrated acceptable reliability and validity for assessing risk among sexual offenders.

Treatment of sexual offenders has been controversial over the years and doubts continue to be raised regarding the effectiveness of treatment for sexual offenders and whether it remains in the appropriate scope of practice for forensic psychologists. However, recent meta-analyses seem to give support for the effectiveness of sexual offender treatment. There also are some components of sexual offender treatment that are generally agreed upon as important, though the empirical support is not clear on any of them being necessary or sufficient. Moreover, it is unclear whether these treatments are effective beyond adult male offenders.

Although adult males have been the predominant focus of the sexual offender literature, there also are a number of other special groups of sexual offenders that may be increasing in prevalence and/or public awareness. Juvenile sexual offenders are the most well studied of these special sexual offender groups with literature indicating the relevant risk factors and some limited information about their treatment. In contrast, much less is known about women who commit sexual crimes. There is some evidence of their prevalence and heterogeneity but little else is known. Research focusing on clergy has appeared even more recently but continues to develop rapidly.

An explosion of legislation has occurred in the United States focusing on the detention and prevention of sexual offenders. Registration and public notification laws require sexual offenders to register with local law enforcement agencies and make the public aware of their presence. Sexual offender residency laws impose limitations on where sexual offenders may live in order to keep them away from individuals perceived to be potential victims. Sexually violent predator (SVP) laws identify a subset of sexual offenders who are the most likely reoffend once released from prison and civilly commit them under the guise of needing additional treatment to reduce their future risk. A number of concerns have been raised about these laws and there therapeutic and anti-therapeutic consequences.

Key Terms

child molester	paraphilia NOS
exhibitionist	pedophile
extrafamilial child molester	penile plethysmograph
frotteurists	relapse prevention
intrafamilial child molester	sexual predator
paraphilia	voyeurs

Further Readings

Marshall, W. L. (2006). Diagnosis and treatment of sexual offenders. In I. B. Weiner & A. K. Hess (Eds.), *The handbook of forensic psychology* (3rd ed., pp. 790–818). Hoboken, NJ: John Wiley & Sons, Inc.

Quinsey, V. L., Harris, G. T., Rice, M. E., & Cormier, C. A. (2006). *Violent offenders: Appraising and managing risk* (2nd ed.). Washington, DC: American Psychological Association.

Insanity is viewed as a legal compromise to a moral dilemma because society believes it is inappropriate for people who do not know what they are doing or cannot control their behavior to be punished. As a result, insanity focuses on an individual's mental state at the time of the criminal act and is often referred to as mental state at the time of the offense or MSO. It is important to remember that insanity refers to someone's mental state at the time of the offense because in Chapter 8, we will discuss competency and the ways in which insanity and competency differ. Competency focuses on someone's mental state during the adjudication process.

One misconception, among many misconceptions that we will discuss in this chapter, is that insanity is a mental illness or is equated with mental illness. Even though the presence of a mental illness or mental defect is central to the different laws that define insanity, insanity is not identical to mental illness. Insanity is a legal term, not a psychological or psychiatric term. You will not find the term insanity listed in the DSM with the diagnostic criteria alongside it as you would other mental illnesses. Someone may suffer from a mental illness and not be insane. Insanity normally requires a level of impairment that is more specific than simply suffering from a mental illness. Moreover, not all mental illnesses are sufficient to establish an insanity defense, as we will discuss later.

Insanity Standards

Part of the controversy surrounding insanity is exemplified in the numerous descriptions or standards of insanity that have existed over time. The intended effects of these changes are another example of therapeutic jurisprudence and the ability of the law to have therapeutic or anti-therapeutic consequences. The definition or standard for insanity has been routinely changed over time because of concern about it being too lenient or sometimes too harsh. There have been continued refinements in hopes that only those people who are truly insane will be acquitted. There are indications that crude standards for insanity date back to at least the thirteenth century in England (Goldstein, Morse, & Shapiro, 2003). However, it was not until the eighteenth century that these crude notions became more formalized.

Wild Beast Standard

One of the first formalized standards of insanity was the **wild beast test**. Early in English common law, a defendant who was believed to be insane was found not guilty but there was not a specific standard for insanity. In 1724, an English judge, Judge Tracy, formally recognized the legal standard that became known as the wild beast standard (*Rex v. Arnold*, 1724) by stating that for someone to be insane he must be totally deprived of his understanding and memory, and not know what he is doing anymore than an infant, a brute, or a wild beast. Such a person should never be punished (Platt & Diamond, 1965). The belief was that someone who was not responsible for his behavior had no more control over his behavior than a wild beast. However, the notion of the wild beast had been around for centuries and was not completely novel to English common law at the time of Tracy's opinion (Platt & Diamond, 1965).

M'Naghten

The wild beast test dominated English law until 1843 and the *M'Naghten* case. The *M'Naghten* case is most frequently identified as the first modern insanity standard. Although "M'Naghten" has been spelled a number of different ways (e.g., McNaughton), we will use the spelling in the original case facts (Goldstein et al., 2003). Daniel M'Naghten appeared to develop a complex delusional belief system that focused on the ruling political party at the time, the Tory Party. M'Naghten believed officials in the Tory Party were out to get him and were going to murder him. He decided to travel to London, kill the Prime Minister and end his own persecution and murder. However, he mistakenly killed the Prime Minister's secretary, Edward Drummond, by shooting him with a pistol (Moran, 1981). M'Naghten's defense team decided to raise an insanity defense. The prosecution agreed that M'Naghten was mentally ill but instead encouraged use of the wild beast test, claiming that his mental illness was not severe enough to justify complete removal of responsibility. Nine expert witnesses testified that M'Naghten was insane because his delusional beliefs made him unable to tell the difference between right and wrong. The judge instructed the jury to find M'Naghten insane and he was committed to a mental hospital for the rest of his life (Verger, 1992).

Public outcry and a reconsideration of the insanity defense is a common result throughout history when a high profile case ends in an insanity verdict (Poulson, Braithwaite, Brondino, & Wuensch, 1997). *M'Naghten* was no different from later instances, except that the outcry was even greater (Freemon, 2001). The public outcry and personal concerns of Queen Victoria, who had received death threats in the past, resulted in a debate in the House of Lords over the use of the insanity defense but ultimately the *M'Naghten* standard was the rule of law (Moran, 1981). The standard states:

> it must be clearly proved that, at the time of the committing of the act, the party accused was labouring under such a defect of reason, from disease of the mind, as not to know the nature and quality of the act he was doing; or, if he did know it, that he did not know he was doing what was wrong. (*M'Naghten* Case, 1843, p. 722)

As with all the modern approaches to insanity, the **M'Naghten standard** first states that the defendant must suffer from a mental illness or "disease of the mind." However, a disease of the mind was not clearly defined at the time and the courts continue to largely ignore a precise definition of mental illness for insanity (Slovenko, 1999; Winick, 1995a). The second prong of *M'Naghten* focuses on the inability to know the nature or quality of the act. This prong is somewhat vague and has two parts, a focus on the *nature* and the *quality* of the act. Courts have interpreted the nature of the acts as pertaining to the physical aspects of the crime. For example, did the defendant know when he placed the poison in his roommate's Red Bull that he would drink it and it would enter his blood stream? Very few defendants fail to meet this requirement of *M'Naghten* (Verger, 1992). The quality of the act suggests that the defendant must know the potential harm that could occur. A very common metaphor used to describe this aspect of *M'Naghten* suggests that a man who chokes a victim believing he was squeezing a lemon would be unable to know the quality of his act. He could not have known that by squeezing a lemon he would be killing a human being.

The third prong of *M'Naghten* focuses on knowing right from wrong. Although this approach was not novel in English law (Zapf, Golding, & Roesch, 2006), it is not completely clear whether the intent was to focus on legal or moral differences. This distinction can be very important, such as in the original trial of Andrea Yates. It was relatively clear that Andrea Yates knew she would be arrested for murdering her children because she called police to report the crime and thereby indicated she knew it was legally wrong. However, it was argued that she believed her actions were morally right because she was saving her children. The original jury decided that Texas law focused on the legality of the act, not the morality of the act, and therefore found her guilty. If Andrea Yates had believed she was only giving her children baths, the question of legal or moral wrong would not have been an issue because she would not have known the nature and the *quality* of the act.

M'Naghten has been criticized as being too narrowly focused or too conservative (Weiner, 1985). *M'Naghten* is normally seen as a more conservative approach to insanity that is likely to result in fewer insanity acquittals than the remaining two modern insanity standards. *M'Naghten* focuses almost exclusively on the cognitive aspects of insanity by emphasizing a defendant's intellectual ability to know and ignores the volitional aspects that could be impaired by a mental illness. Volitional refers to a person's ability to choose a given course of action. An insanity standard that considers volition would generally recognize problems with impulse control.

Despite this narrow focus, *M'Naghten* was widely adopted across the United States, though it was challenged early because of its narrow focus (Zapf et al., 2006). Several states began to reconsider the narrow focus of *M'Naghten* and included an **irresistible impulse test** with it after the initial adoption of the standard. The irresistible impulse test normally suggests that even if a defendant knows the nature and quality of an act and is aware that it is wrong, he may be unable to stop his behavior. For example, assume that Mikey has been suffering from command hallucinations telling him to purchase ceramic lawn gnomes to protect his house from intruders. Mikey may resist the voices because he does not have any money in his checking account and cannot afford the lawn gnomes. He knows it would be wrong to write the check without sufficient funds but suppose the voices overpower him and he is unable to resist the urge to purchase the lawn gnomes from the Home Shopping Network. In this instance, the defendant could qualify as insane under the irresistible impulse test. A law review article at the time, noted that *M'Naghten* had either been fully adopted, altered to include some mention of an irresistible impulse test, or been replaced by a new standard, the product rule, by the early 1900s (Crotty, 1924).

M'Naghten continues to be the most prominent standard for insanity in the United States in some form. Reviews of the relevant state laws suggest that some version of *M'Naghten* is the insanity standard in about half the states. The Canadian insanity defense states that a defendant can be found insane if he or she is suffering from a mental disorder that resulted in his or her failure to understand the nature of the act or to know that it was wrong (as cited in Viljoen, Roesch, Ogloff, & Zapf, 2003). This standard appears very similar to the standard used in most jurisdictions in the United States (Viljoen et al., 2003). Nonetheless, there are two other significant insanity standards that have been and continue to be used in the United States.

We can start to see some of the potential scope of practice issues for forensic psychologists in this first of the modern insanity standards. Forensic psychologists should be able to evaluate the presence of a mental illness. It is one of the key aspects of their training (see Chapter 2). However, are they capable of doing so retrospectively, days or months after a crime has been committed and the defendant is now medicated or had time to recover from their previous psychological difficulties? We have talked about forensic psychologists determining someone's cognitive abilities like intelligence and memory. However, are forensic psychologists able to take those abilities and determine if someone knew the difference between right and wrong or knew what they were doing? Are they able to do so in a way that conforms to precise legal wording? These are important questions in discussing the remaining standards. They are also probably questions without a definitive answer but they are important to keep in mind now and in our later discussion regarding the reliability and validity of insanity evaluations.

The Product Rule and *Durham*

An 1869 New Hampshire case first established use of the so called **product rule** (*State v. Pike*, 1869). This standard is referred to as the product rule because the court declined the more complex approach specified in *M'Naghten* in favor of finding a person insane if the crime "was the offspring or product of mental disease in the defendant" (*State v. Pike*, 1869, p. 442). In 1954, the United States Court of Appeals in the District of Columbia adopted the product rule and it became known as the **Durham rule**. In *Durham v. United States* (1954), Monte Durham was charged with "housebreaking and petit larceny" and pled insanity (Weiner, 1985, p. 9). The influential Judge Bazelon (the same judge who later presided in *Jenkins*) wrote the court's opinion and stated that experts should be of GBMI decrease the number of NGRI verdicts but it also decreased the number of guilty verdicts. Roberts, Golding, and Fincham (1987) further clarified this point by confirming that the addition of the GBMI alternative reduces the number of defendants found NGRI in cases exhibiting severe mental illness, and it reduces the number of defendants found guilty in cases of milder forms of mental illness. Therefore, it appears that the addition of the GBMI verdict choice can cause a verdict shift both from NGRI to GBMI and from guilty to GBMI depending on case specifics. Overall, the results clearly indicate that the presence of an additional verdict option in the form of GBMI influences jurors' decisions (Poulson, Wuensch, & Brondino, 1998). Whether jurors' selection of the GBMI verdict is due to the appropriateness of the verdict or the mere fact that it is an alternative verdict (i.e., a verdict other than guilty, not guilty, or NGRI) is unclear at this time.

Insanity Myths

As the previous section examining the influence of the different insanity standards seemed to suggest, there are a number of misconceptions regarding the insanity defense (Perlin, 1996). These misconceptions or myths typically focus on the overuse of the defense, severity of crimes at issue in these cases, severity of the mental illnesses involved, the disposition of insanity acquittees, and the dangerousness of insanity acquittees. The belief that the standard of insanity makes a significant difference in the rate of acquittals has been the focus of much of the public and legislative attention. This belief is based on the idea that the insanity defense is overused and abused by defendants. However, the available evidence suggests a very different picture. Though the rates vary between different jurisdictions, studies suggest that the insanity defense is rarely raised and even more rarely results in an acquittal. On average, the insanity defense appears to be raised in about 1% of all felony cases and only successful about 26% of the time (Cirincione, Steadman, & McGreevy, 1995). However, there is significant variability and results are rarely comprehensive. For example, studies have been able to obtain usable data from 5, 7, 8, and 10 states respectively and have been largely confined to the most populous counties in those states (Callahan, Steadman, McGreevy, & Robbins, 1991; Cirincione et al., 1995; McGinley & Pasewark, 1989; Pasewark & McGinley, 1985). Furthermore, these rates vary dramatically between states because of a number of unique differences in the procedures and laws. For example Callahan et al. (1991) found that insanity plea rates varied anywhere from 0.30% to 5.74% of felonies cases and the acquittal rates varied anywhere from 7.3% to 87% in one state where it appeared that insanity pleas were largely entered via a plea arrangement between the prosecution and defense.

The 1% rate of insanity pleas and 26% of those ending in an acquittal are in clear contrast to the public perception (Silver, Cirincione, & Steadman, 1994). Table 7.2 shows these comparisons. Furthermore, there is a negative

Table 7.2.   Public Beliefs and the Actual Insanity Defense

	Perception	Actual
Use of the insanity defense		
Percentage of insanity pleas	37%	1%
Percentage of insanity acquittals	44%	26%
Disposition of acquittees		
Percentage sent to mental hospital	51%	85%
Percentage freed	26%	15%
Conditional release		12%
Outpatient		3%
Release		1%
Length of confinement		
All crimes	22 months	33 months
Murder	–	76 months

Source: Adapted from Table 2 of Silver, Cirincione, & Steadman (1994)

relationship between frequency of an insanity plea and the success ($r = -.67$) (Cirincione et al., 1995) so defendants in states that use the defense more frequently are less successful. It is clear that the public significantly overestimates both the use and the success of the insanity defense but it may be possible to alter these beliefs. In one study, about 92% of community respondents believed the insanity defense was over used but if educated about the actual rates, only 52% believed it was over used (Jeffrey & Pasewark, 1983). These data seem to suggest that much of the public concern over the insanity defense is due to a lack of knowledge about actual rates of use and success.

A second common misconception is that insanity acquittees are not severely mentally ill. In a study of over 1,700 pretrial defendants from federal courts, results found that 77% of those found insane were suffering from psychosis, a mood disorder, mental retardation, or an organic disorder and only 1% were malingering mental illness (Cochrane, Grisso, & Frederick, 2001). Callahan et al. (1991) found that almost 70% of insanity acquittees were diagnosed with some form of psychosis, an additional 16% suffered other major mental illnesses, and 4.8% were mentally retarded. Cirincione et al. (1995) further demonstrated that those individuals who suffered from a major mental illness were significantly more likely to be found insane than those without a major mental illness. Research also indicates that the vast majority of insanity acquittees have been previously hospitalized for mental health reasons (Callahan et al., 1991) and at least one previous hospitalization was related to a successful insanity acquittal (Cirincione et al., 1995). Again, results suggest that public perception is inaccurate and that those who plea and are acquitted on the basis of insanity are severely mentally ill.

Evaluations of Insanity

Of all the different legal questions that forensic psychologists seek to assist the courts on, insanity investigations are among the more difficult for several reasons. First, the legal doctrine tends to be unclear. The nature of mental illness sufficient for insanity acquittals has been largely undefined by the courts. Furthermore, there have not been clear answers to whether knowing the difference between right and wrong should emphasize a legal distinction, a moral distinction or the level of impairment. Second, forensic evaluations are retrospective and require the forensic psychologist to reconstruct a defendant's mental state weeks or even months after the crime. This task often proves difficult because psychological assessment methods assess current mental health, they do not allow the evaluator to travel back in time to assess someone's mental state precisely during the crime. Because of the retrospective nature of insanity evaluations, there also must be a greater reliance on third party information. Although psychological measures do not allow for retrospective examinations, assessments of current mental functioning along with consultation with police reports, witnesses, and other prior records begin to offer a picture of most defendants. Fourth, there are no universally accepted interviews or psychological tests for insanity evaluations. Although we will discuss the two specialized forensic tests used by some experts for this purpose, there is a great deal of variability in forensic psychologists' approaches to insanity evaluations and they may exhibit less than ideal reliability as a result. Despite the challenges involved in conducting insanity evaluations, there are some common recommendations (Borum, 2003b; Goldstein et al., 2003; Melton, Petrila, Poythress, & Slobogin, 1997; Rogers & Shuman, 2000a; Zapf et al., 2006).

Common Procedures for Insanity Evaluations

Insanity evaluations tend to consist of three major components similar to most forensic assessments: an interview, use of forensic related assessment instruments, and collection of third party and collateral information (Zapf et al., 2006). However, there are not well-established and empirically validated comprehensive approaches to conducting an insanity evaluation. Borum and Grisso (1996) surveyed forensic psychologists and psychiatrists asking about the elements central to an insanity report. Results revealed eleven different elements essential for a report: 1) psychiatric history; 2) current mental status; 3) formal mental status exam; 4) any current psychotropic medication; 5) psychological testing; 6) mental health records; 7) police information; 8) presence or absence of any prior diagnosis; 9) presence/absence and degree of any alcohol/substance abuse; 10) defendant's description of the offense; and 11) collateral description of the offense. Nonetheless, there is some evidence for the overall reliability and validity of insanity evaluations and some of the assessment approaches commonly utilized.

Reliability and Validity of Insanity Evaluations

There is little empirical information regarding the methods used in insanity evaluations. Research has generally suggested that mental health professionals rarely find a defendant insane, in contrast again with the public sentiment. Cochrane et al. (2001) found that only 12% of 719 referrals for insanity were found insane in a federal sample of offenders. In examining the decisions of clinicians, Murrie and Warren (2005) noted that most clinicians found between 5% and 25% of their insanity referrals insane. Mental health professionals also vary the percentage of insanity decisions according to the different standards in place, unlike the jurors who frequently decide these cases (Wettstein, Mulvey, & Rogers, 1991). Finally, the most important factor in insanity findings may be the ultimate decision of the expert (Steadman, Keitner, Braff, & Arvanties, 1983). As a result, it is very important to assess the reliability and validity of these decisions.

An examination of the reliability and validity of insanity evaluations is especially important because of the nature of the adversarial process. Brodsky (1991) and Rogers (1987) warned of the potential for forensic psychologists and other mental health professionals to become committed to a particular legal outcome or unintentionally mold their evaluation to the theory of the retaining attorney. Otto (1989) conducted an analogue study in which he examined the potential source of bias in insanity cases and found that expert testimony in these cases may vary according to the side that retained the expert. Advanced graduate students in a clinical psychology program were more likely to rate the defendant as guilty if retained by the prosecution and more likely to rate the defendant as NGRI if retained by the defense. However, this study used graduate students, not forensic psychologists or other fully trained mental health professionals, and the sample was small ($n = 32$). Beckham, Annis, and Gustafson (1989) did not find any bias attributable to the side that retained them among 180 forensic experts who evaluated a set of hypothetical case materials. However, Homant & Kennedy (1987) also found that in three separate studies, experts' political beliefs were related to their ultimate conclusions in a hypothetical insanity case.

Studies focusing on the reliability between raters have found high rates of agreement between them. Fukunaga, Pasewark, Hawkins, and Gudeman (1981) were able to examine 355 official cases in Hawaii. Courts typically appointed two independent evaluators to assess an insanity defendant. Examining these records, they found a 92% rate of agreement between the evaluators. However, it was unclear whether independent professionals communicated with one another prior to writing the report, potentially increasing the rate of agreement if they did collaborate. Overall, these high rates of agreement should not be surprising given that insanity verdicts are usually the result of an agreement between the defense and prosecution and rarely involve a trial and a battle of the experts (Melton et al., 1997). The cases that are likely to involve a contested trial are the ones that are less likely to involve clear cases either way and involve a host of unique characteristics likely to reduce consensus among experts (Zapf et al., 2006). These studies also tend to focus on overall agreement and do not look at the different characteristics that relate to an expert's final decision. One study that did examine the interrater reliability of one of these characteristics, diagnostic symptoms, found a significant agreement between forensic experts ($r = .73$) who were given a set of ambiguous case materials designed to produce the least agreement (Beckham et al., 1989). They also examined the characteristics that related to guilty and NGRI decisions by the experts. Those experts who found the defendant guilty rated the defendant as displaying less schizophrenia at the time of the offense, judged the defendant's behavior as less likely a product of the mental illness, considered third party information as more important, rated the clinical interview and some of the cognitive assessment data presented as less important, and had greater forensic experience (Beckham et al., 1989).

It is also problematic to study the validity of insanity evaluations because of the lack of a criterion measure or gold standard (Borum, 2003b). Typically, the decision of the evaluators is compared to the final verdict in these cases. However, the final verdict is influenced by the expert opinion and therefore the criterion of the final verdict is biased in favor of the validity of these decisions. Not surprisingly, there is high agreement between the final verdicts in insanity cases and the judgments of the involved experts. Fukunaga et al. (1981) found 93% agreement between the expert conclusions and the final judgment. In a study of 143 defendants who pled the equivalent of NGRI in a metropolitan county for one year, there was 98% agreement between the evaluating experts opinion on the final verdict (Janofsky, Vandewalle, & Rappeport, 1989). The high rates of agreement also suggest that the so called battle of experts is not the norm in insanity cases (Janofsky et al., 1989).

Forensic Assessment Instruments

In order to improve upon the reliability and validity of forensic assessments, standard practice appears to be moving toward the use of forensic assessment instruments (Zapf et al., 2006). However, there appear to be only two specialized instruments available for use in assessments of insanity. Moreover, the reliability and validity of both of these instruments has been questioned and significant caution encouraged in using either instrument. (Melton et al., 1997; Rogers & Shuman, 2000b).

The Mental State at the Time of the Offense Screening Evaluation (MSE; Slobogin, Melton, & Showalter, 1984) is a semi-structured screening measure to asses issues related to criminal responsibility, such as insanity. It consists of three sections that focus on historical information assessing a defendant's prior psychological and cognitive functioning, offense related information, and information about the defendant's current mental status. There are not any published studies in regard to the reliability of the MSE and the only indication of its validity is in the original article introducing the measure. The original study examined the decisions of 24 experts who evaluated three defendants in teams of two. Results of the original study suggested the instrument was able to screen out those individuals who were obviously insane and not in need of any further evaluation (Slobogin et al., 1984). However, the MSE has been criticized for a lack of additional research and that it should not be used as a sole determinant of insanity, if at all (Poythress, Melton, Petrila, & Slobogin, 2000; Rogers & Shuman, 2000b), despite earlier recommendations for expanding its use (Melton et al., 1997). A recent review of the instrument has concluded that the instrument can be used as one piece of a comprehensive insanity evaluation (Zapf et al., 2006).

The evidence supporting the use of the Rogers Criminal Responsibility Assessment Scales (R-CRAS; Rogers, 1984) is a little more abundant than the MSE. The R-CRAS is a 30 item measure intended to be used to standardize the information obtained from an insanity evaluation. Specifically, the R-CRAS was designed with the ALI criteria but the author also recommends its use in jurisdictions using the *M'Naghten* standard. It also has items relating to GBMI verdict alternative (Rogers & Shuman, 2000a). The 30 items are divided into 5 components: patient's reliability, organicity, psychopathology, cognitive control, and behavioral control (Borum, 2003b). The R-CRAS does not dictate that information on any of the relevant items be collected in a particular order or according to a specific set of questions. It is intended to be a tool to quantify or standardize insanity evaluations. Conclusions on the major criteria are then used to derive either a sane, insane, or no opinion overall conclusion. Though the interrater reliability for individual items is somewhat low, the 5 components demonstrate good reliability (Borum, 2003b). The summary ratings obtained from the R-CRAS also exhibit high rates of agreement (93–97%) with independent rater final decisions (Borum, 2003b). However, the R-CRAS has been criticized for the way in which it measures some of the items, emphasis on the ultimate issue, the quantification of judgment areas that are "logical and/or intuitive in nature" (p. 234), and unsupported scientific rigor (Melton et al., 1997). Rogers and Shuman (2000a) have accepted and addressed these criticisms but ultimately seem to correctly conclude that the R-CRAS is better than any alternative and represents a significant step forward in the assessment of insanity, if used as part of a comprehensive evaluation.

Malingering and Insanity

Despite the use of some specialized measures for insanity evaluations, many people claim that insanity is easily malingered (Golding, 1992a, see Figure 7.1). Box 7.2 gives one famous example of an attempt to malinger by the Hillside Strangler. Given the secondary gain involved in insanity evaluations, the presence of malingering should always be considered. However, there is insufficient evidence to conclude that insanity acquittees are successfully feigning mental illness or neuropsychological impairments at significant rates. Cochrane et al.

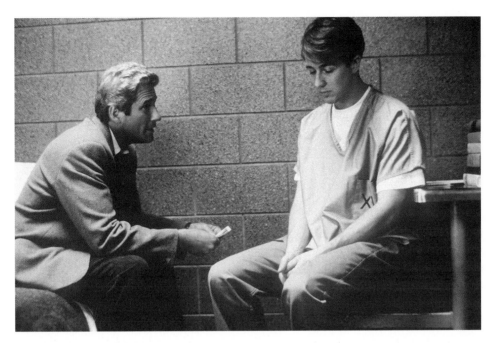

Figure 7.1   *Primal Fear* is a 1996 movie in which Ed Norton malingers dissociative identity disorder in order to be found insane for the murder of a priest. Richard Gere plays his attorney who is also initially fooled by him. © Paramount / The Kobal Collection / Ron Phillips

(2001) identified only one individual in over 700 federal insanity referrals that was diagnosed with malingering, though more subtle exaggeration and defensiveness are likely. Nonetheless, forensic experts should remain on alert for potential signs of malingering such as those identified in Chapter 2. There also are a number of standardized measures designed to assess for the presence of malingering. Some measures mentioned in Chapter 2 are arguably better (SIRS) than others (MMPI-2) in the detection of malingered psychopathology. Forensic psychologists should also make sure to focus on both the exaggeration of psychopathology and cognitive and neuropsychological impairments with standardized measures (Rogers & Shuman, 2000a). Rogers and Shuman (2005) even go so far as to say that expert testimony on malingering that does not involve a standardized measure, probably does not fulfill the *Daubert* criteria discussed in Chapter 3.

Other Issues of Criminal Responsibility

Besides insanity, there are a number of additional issues related to criminal responsibility that include automatism, diminished capacity, and intoxication. In each of these instances, there is a negation of mens rea, a term we discussed

Box 7.2.   A Lesson Regarding Insanity and Malingering: The Hillside Strangler

Kenneth Bianchi and his cousin, Angelo Buono, were dubbed the *Hillside Strangler* after a series of rapes and murders of young women in the Los Angeles area during 1977 and early 1978. Victims were typically raped, tortured, and strangled to death with their bodies often being dumped on hillsides around Los Angeles. The media and law enforcement originally suspected it was only one killer and it was not until well into the investigation that law enforcement officials realized it was likely two men. After he was apprehended, Bianchi decided to plead insanity based on the belief that he suffered form multiple personality disorder or as it is now called, dissociative identity disorder. He reportedly got the idea from the movie *Sybil* and called his altered personality who killed the women, Steve Walker.

Though two experts originally believed Bianchi suffered from dissociative identity disorder, two additional experts concluded that Bianchi was faking, or malingering, the disorder. There were several indications that Bianchi was malingering the disorder.

One clue was uncovered by the police when they discovered that Bianchi had used the name of a student, Steve Walker, to obtain a college diploma fraudulently so he could practice psychology. Also, while Bianchi was pretending to be Steve Walker he slipped several times and referred to Steve as "he" instead of "I." In addition, Dr. Martin Orne was able to trick Bianchi during his clinical interview of him. Dr. Orne was an expert in determining whether people were truly hypnotized and during his attempt to hypnotize Bianchi he determined that Bianchi met several criteria for someone who is actually not hypnotized. Orne also purposely mislead Bianchi by telling him that people who suffer from dissociative identity disorder have more than one additional personality. Soon after an additional personality named Bill surfaced, with two others soon following. Eventually, Bianchi agreed to testify against Buono, though he was very uncooperative during the trial itself. He is now serving multiple life sentences.

earlier. The negation of mens rea leads to a reduction in criminal responsibility but normally not a complete excuse for it. Empirical support for forensic practice in these areas is even more sparse than for insanity defenses (Clark, 2006). The role of the forensic psychologist continues to be similar in terms of the assessment of a defendant's mental state at the time of a given crime, though the application of that expertise to more ambiguous legal notions becomes even more complex and more difficult.

Automatism recognizes there are criminal acts that may occur involuntarily. Traditional examples typically include a defendant who lacks full consciousness because she is sleeping, experienced a head injury, or suffers from epilepsy or dissociation. There tend to be three differences between insanity and automatism (Melton et al., 1997). Insanity requires a mental illness and automatism does not. For example, the defendant could be sleeping. The prosecution typically has the burden of negating automatism defense whereas the defense has

Table 8.1.   Comparison of Insanity and Competency

Insanity	Competency
Focus on mental state at time of the offense	Focus on mental state at any point along the adjudication process
Requires presence of mental illness	Mental illness not required
Legal defense to criminal charges	Postpones adjudication process
Requires admission of crime	Does not require admission

of incompetence leads to a postponement in the legal proceeding. For example, a defendant who is found incompetent to stand trial is not simply released but is more likely to be referred to a mental health facility in order to restore his or her competency and then face trial once competency is restored. Third, the standards for competency and insanity are vastly different. Insanity requires the presence of a mental illness. Although the threshold for competency involves a defendant's mental state, most competency standards do not require the presence of a mental illness, even though most of those found incompetent suffer from a mental illness. Fourth, a competency evaluation does not require a defendant admit to committing the crime. Defendants must only know the meaning of the charges and the consequences of their actions at any point in the process to be competent (Gutheil, 1999). In fact, a report focused solely on competence typically does not include any statements made by the defendant concerning the crime (Sales, Miller, & Hall, 2005). These distinctions should help keep the two issues separate throughout the rest of the chapter (see Table 8.1 for a summary).

Competency to Stand Trial (CST)

Our discussion of competency will focus, not only on criminal competency but more precisely on competency to stand trial (CST). Competency to stand trial is the most prominent and frequently examined aspect of criminal competency. Some argue that CST should serve as a "blueprint" for research and practice in other competency areas that have been less frequently examined (Zapf, Viljoen, Whittemore, Poythress, & Roesch, 2002, p. 171). Moreover, legal rulings have suggested that the legal standard for competency to stand trial should be equated with other instances in which competency arises (*Godinez v. Moran*, 1993; *Regina v. Whittle*, 1994).

There is a long history in English common law of stopping legal proceedings because defendants were incompetent to stand trial. Stafford (2003) states that this notion traces back further to the prohibition against trials **in absentia**. A defendant could not be absent for his own trial (i.e., in absentia). This practice evolved from the need to be physically present for one's trial into the requirement to be mentally present at the time of trial. Statutes and case law have continued to refine these early notions that emphasized the competence of a defendant in order to ensure the fairness and accuracy of the legal proceedings. The Canadian standard for competency, or **fitness** as it is frequently termed, defines someone who is unfit to stand trial as someone who is unable to understand the nature or unable to object to the proceedings, unable to understand the consequences of the proceedings, or communicate with counsel. However, the Canadian standard specifically requires the inabilities be the result of a mental disorder. The dominant standard in the United States is based on the Supreme Court ruling in *Dusky v. United States* (1960). *Dusky* required that a defendant exhibit "sufficient present ability to consult with his lawyer with a reasonable degree of rational understanding – and whether he has a rational as well as factual understanding of the proceedings against him" (p. 402). It does not specifically require a mental illness (Cruise & Rogers, 1998) though most defendants found incompetent suffer from severe mental illness. Competency has been further defined by the federal courts (*Wieter v. Settle*, 1961) and by specific states (e.g., *State v. Guatney*, 1980). The notions of competency in the United States and Canada are similar but the U.S. standard tends to result in a higher threshold for competency in the United States (Zapf & Roesch, 2001).

Prevalence of CST

Estimates suggest that as many as 60,000 competency evaluations take place each year in the United States (Bonnie & Grisso, 2000) and that this figure has consistently risen from 25,000 over two decades ago (Steadman, Monahan, Harstone, Davis, & Robbins, 1982). Estimates vary but pretrial competency evaluations appear to occur in 2–8% of all felony cases (Hoge, Bonnie, Poythress, & Monahan, 1992). Attorneys further have doubts about their client's competence in as many as 15% of all felony cases with less frequent doubts in misdemeanor cases (Hoge et al., 1997), but only obtain competency evaluations in half of these instances (Poythress, Bonnie, Hoge, Monahan, & Oberlander, 1994). Attorneys routinely refer to the low threshold for competence (i.e., it is easy to be found competent, difficult to be found incompetent) as one of the reasons for not obtaining more competency evaluations and often cite client passivity and rejection of the attorney's advice as reasons for originally doubting competency (Hoge et al., 1992; Poythress et al., 1994). Ultimately, only about 20% of defendants referred for competency evaluations are deemed incompetent (Zapf et al., 2006). CST evaluations are the most frequently occurring forensic evaluation in the legal system (Warren et al., 2006) and more money is spent on the evaluation, adjudication, and treatment of people with suspected competency issues than any other forensic issue (Golding, 1992b).

Procedures in CST

Though procedures vary from jurisdiction to jurisdiction, there are some generally universal procedures involved in CST evaluations. A defendant is legally presumed to be competent unless an issue of competency is raised (Bullock, 2003). Anyone can raise the issue of competency but normally it is the defense attorney that raises the issue because it is in the best interest of the defendant. However, the trial judge is obligated to raise the issue if there is any doubt about the defendant's competency (*Pate v. Robinson*, 1966). This determination can be based on irrational behavior, demeanor at trial, or expert opinion (*Drope v. Missouri*, 1975). Wulach (1980) identified several reasons for ensuring competency. First, a competent defendant increases the accuracy of the trial because the defendant is able to communicate the facts of the case. Second, in order to ensure fairness and the defendant's due process, the defendant must be allowed to exercise his full rights. Third, the integrity of the process can be questioned for legal as well as moral reasons if incompetent defendants are tried. Fourth, the purpose of punishment is not upheld if a defendant is convicted and does not understand the meaning or intent of the punishment. In addition to these intentional reasons for ensuring the competency of the defendant, some commentators argue that competency is increasingly being used for trial strategy purposes. For example, a competency issue may be raised to avoid a trial or avoid a legal sanction and instead have the defendant committed to a mental health hospital instead of serving prison time (Slovenko, 1995).

Once a competency evaluation is identified as necessary and the evaluation is completed, a report is submitted to the court. At this point, a hearing may be scheduled to further examine the findings of the report and allow the forensic psychologist who conducted the evaluation to testify. However, these hearings are normally very brief and they rarely occur (Zapf et al., 2006). In most instances, all the involved parties stipulate to the findings of the report.

If the parties stipulate the defendant is competent, the process continues toward trial. If the defendant is incompetent, there are several possible outcomes. The trial may be delayed until the defendant's competency is restored. Restoration may take place through a variety of psychiatric, psychological, and psychoeducational approaches that I will describe later. However, there are limits on the amount of time that a defendant can be held while awaiting restoration of competency. In *Jackson v. Indiana* (1972) the United States Supreme Court ruled that a defendant can only be institutionalized for a reasonable period of time to determine if the defendant can be restored to competency in the foreseeable future (Box 8.1). If the defendant is not institutionalized in order to restore competency, the charges can be dismissed with the option that the prosecution may file them again in the future. In either case, the defendant also may face civil commitment, whether it is eventually determined that they cannot be restored to competency in the foreseeable future or if the charges are to be dismissed.

Competency Evaluations

At the heart of the legal process is the competency evaluation itself. Much like in insanity evaluations, there appears to be significant agreement between the

Box 8.1.   Importance of Jackson v. Indiana (1972)

Jackson v. Indiana (1972) was a Supreme Court case that clearly intended to improve the therapeutic outcome associated with the institutionalization of incompetent defendants. Prior to *Jackson*, defendants who had been found incompetent to stand trial could be held indefinitely no matter how trivial their alleged crime. Theon Jackson was a 27 year-old, deaf mute who could not read or write and had almost no ability to communicate. He was originally charged with two purse snatchings in 1968 that totaled about $9 worth of property. Prior to trial he was evaluated by two different mental health experts and found to be incompetent to stand trial because his mental retardation and inability to communicate would make him unable to understand the nature of the proceedings or participate in his defense. Because his disabilities were not treatable, this finding amounted to a life sentence for Jackson.

This practice was not uncommon at the time, as many incompetent defendants were confined to state hospitals for years and were more likely to die in the facility than ever be released.

However, the purpose of competency was to ensure fairness and it did not seem fair to hand a man a life sentence for stealing two purses. As a result, the United States Supreme Court held that Jackson's due process rights were violated because of the failure to obtain a speedy trial and his continued incarceration without any criminal charges or conviction against him. The Court ordered that he either had to be released or civilly committed after he was held for a reasonable period of time. The Court did not further define a reasonable period of time but it has often been equated with the amount of time a defendant would otherwise serve if convicted of the original crime.

judge's final determination of competency and the expert's evaluation (Zapf, Hubbard, Cooper, Wheeles, & Ronan, 2004). However, there is no standard approach for conducting competency evaluations and there appears to be a great deal of variability. Borum & Grisso (1995) surveyed forensic psychologists and psychiatrists regarding their standard practice in conducting competence to stand trial evaluations. They found that forensic psychologists were evenly split on the importance of using psychological testing with 51% seeing testing as essential and 49% viewing it as optional. These forensic psychologists also mentioned they used objective measures of personality (90%), neuropsychological testing (42%), competency instruments (36%) and projective tests (33%). Heilbrun & Collins (1995) examined the CST reports themselves to assess standard practice in these evaluations. They found that 15.3% of the reports included mention of psychological testing with the MMPI and the Wechsler Adult Intelligence Scale-Revised (WAIS-R) as the most frequently used. Lally (2003) found that among forensic psychologists with greater expertise, 62% recommended use of the current version of the WAIS and 56% recommended a specific forensic measure of competency (e.g., MacArthur Competence Assessment Tool – Criminal Adjudication; MacCAT-CA).

Table 8.2. Frequency of Use in Competency Evaluations

Method	Percentage used
Clinical interview	85–100
Mental status exam	45–93
Psychological tests	9–69
Review of collateral information	0–96
Competency specific tests	0–25

Source: Nicholson and Norwood (2000)

Nicholson and Norwood (2000) reviewed the available studies and found the percentage of experts who reported using a different method varied with 85–100% reporting use of a clinical interview, 45–93% reporting use of a mental status exam, 9–69% reported use of psychological tests, and 0–25% reported use of competency specific forensic instruments (See Table 8.2). Although the composition of the samples and whether forensic psychiatrists were included with the forensic psychologists (psychiatrists are not typically trained in the administration of psychological tests) might be a plausible explanation for the reduced rates of test usage and the variability, Nicholson and Norwood (2000) concluded that it did not explain all the variability. Rates also varied across studies for review of collateral information with anywhere from 0% to 96% of the experts using review of records (Nicholson & Norwood, 2000). They generally concluded that there does not appear to be a consistent standard of practice among forensic psychologists conducting CST evaluations.

Competency Measures

Unlike insanity evaluations, there are over half a dozen specialized forensic measures designed to assess competency to stand trial (Zapf & Viljoen, 2003). Furthermore, even though specialized tests are not used in the majority of competency evaluations the continued development of these measures marks an important step forward in the development of standardized competency evaluations (Zapf et al., 2002). The available instruments reflect a range of methods from self-report questionnaires to interview-based instruments. The use of standardized forensic instruments specifically focused on competency to stand trial is in keeping with trends in the field of forensic psychology.

The first two attempts at a systematic measure to assess competency were the Competency Screening Test (CST; Lipsitt, Lelos, & McGarry, 1971) and the Competency to Stand Trial Assessment Instrument (CAI; McGarry, 1973). The CAI is a 13-item measure that identifies 13 functions related to competency that can be assessed through two or three interview questions. It has been largely criticized for a lack of norms and scoring criteria and some of the assumptions it is based upon (Cruise & Rogers, 1998). The CST is a

22-item sentence completion questionnaire that was developed as a screening instrument and consists of items such as, "If the jury finds me guilty, I ___." Each item is scored according to the level of competency exhibited in the response (0 for an incompetent response, 1 for a fairly competent response, and 2 for a competent response). The instrument exhibits good reliability but high false positive rates or tends to classify a number of people as incompetent who are competent (Nicholson, Robertson, Johnson, & Jensen, 1988). As a result, the measure has largely been unstudied over the past decade (Stafford, 2003).

Another measure of competency that has been developed and revised from its original version is the Georgia Court Competency Test – Mississippi Version Revised (GCCT-MSH). The GCCT originally included 17 items that focused on courtroom and legal practices, current charges and likely consequences, and the defendant's relationship with his attorney (Wildman et al., 1978). The GCCT was revised and now includes 21 items devised to screen out defendants who are clearly competent to stand trial. Defendants are asked to visually identify different aspects of the courtroom and then respond to a series of interview questions. Although the instrument exhibits good reliability and validity (Nicholson, Briggs, & Robertson, 1988), the GCCT and GCCT-MSH have been criticized because they focus on foundational competencies (e.g., the ability to communicate with one's attorney and the nature of the charges) instead of the decisional competences (i.e., overall cognitive ability) found in other competency measures (Zapf & Viljoen, 2003).

The Fitness Interview Test (FIT; Roesch, Webster, & Eaves, 1984) and the Fitness Interview Test – Revised (FIT-R; Roesch, Zapf, Eaves, & Webster, 1998) are structured interviews based on Canadian law. They are similar to the Interdisciplinary Fitness Interview (IFI; Golding, Roesch, & Schreiber, 1984) which is based on U.S. law. The FIT and FIT-R consist of items designed to assess psychopathology and the legal issues involved in competency. Questions are divided into specific areas: the ability to understand the nature of the proceedings, the ability to understand the potential consequences, and the ability to communicate with one's attorney. Research has supported the use of the FIT and FIT-R in terms of the reliability and validity (Viljoen, Roesch, & Zapf, 2002; Zapf & Roesch, 1997).

The MacArthur Foundation Research Network developed the most recent instruments that resemble the state of the art in competency measures: the MacArthur Structured Assessment of the Competencies of Criminal defendants (MacSAD-CD; Hoge et al., 1997) and the MacArthur Competence Assessment Tool – Criminal Adjudication (MacCAT-CA; Poythress et al., 1999). MacSAD-CD was originally developed to distinguish competent from incompetent defendants and to distinguish the dynamic nature of competency among distinct quantifiable domains (Hoge et al., 1997). Research found it was positively related to clinical judgments of competency and negatively related to psychopathology and cognitive deficits (Stafford, 2003). However, the MacSAD-CD was difficult to administer for clinical purposes and therefore the authors created a modified version, the MacCAT-CA. The MacCAT-CA emphasizes three different areas of competence: understanding, reasoning and appreciation. Early indications are that the MacCAT-CA is sound in terms of its reliability and validity (Zapf, Skeem, & Golding, 2005). However, there are several items that utilize a hypothetical case vignette that may not apply directly to the vast majority of cases (Rogers, Grandjean, Tillbook, Vitacco, & Sewell, 2001; Zapf et al., 2005). This aspect of the instrument would limit its generalizability.

Research has consistently demonstrated that across different competency instruments, incompetent defendants perform more poorly (Hoge et al., 1996; Nicholson & Kugler, 1991). However, there are some special considerations in using these instruments. Because of the low threshold for finding a defendant competent, it is important to have instruments that allow experts to quickly screen out potential defendants that clearly will meet the low threshold (Zapf & Viljoen, 2003). Although these measures allow for a standardized approach that is likely to lead to more reliable results, relying on a single measure without consideration of the contextual issues may hamper their use in individualized assessments of competency (Zapf & Viljoen, 2003). As a result, it would be unadvisable for a practicing forensic psychologist to simply base a decision of competence on a score on one of these single measures.

A comprehensive approach to competency evaluations

Beyond the use of specific measures of intelligence, psychopathology, or even specialized forensic instruments, is the consideration of a general approach to competency assessment. Many have argued that forensic psychologists often are misguided in their approach to addressing legal questions related to competency (Winick, 1995b). Grisso (1988) argues for the clear understanding of the legal notion of competency and where it diverges from related psychological constructs. He further identifies five objectives that allow for the translation of "the legal definition and procedure of competency to stand trial into objectives for competency evaluations" (Grisso, 1988, p. 11). Grisso (1988) argues that competency evaluations should include a *functional* description of specific abilities, a *causal* explanation for deficits in competency abilities, the *interactive* significance of deficits in competency abilities, *conclusory* opinions about legal competency and incompetency, and *prescriptive* remediation for deficits in competency abilities.

It is important to focus on the defendant's **functional abilities** by examining her strengths and weaknesses as they apply to the legal standard. Instead of a forensic psychologist focusing on general abilities such as intelligence and mental illness, the forensic psychologist should describe the relationship of these general abilities and their impact on a defendant's ability to communicate with an attorney, understand the legal proceedings, or describe the inability to do so during the trial because of any deficits. The *causal* objective encourages the forensic psychologist to explain the basis for any of the functional deficits previously identified. The basis for these deficits are normally mental illness but also may be related to a lack of awareness or low education about the legal process, or situational determinants like fatigue or malingering (Grisso, 1988). The *interactive* objective encourages an identification of the specific aspects of the trial that may impact the functional difficulties. This objective takes into consideration that two defendants with identical abilities may exhibit different levels of competency, given the nature of their different trials. One defendant may be on trial for a minor theft, facing only probation, and have a number of independent witnesses that will testify to guilt. Another defendant may be on trial for murder and the only witness able to describe the events of the murder. The level of stress involved for the murder defendant may cause his functioning to significantly deteriorate during his trial, while the other defendant will have little trouble. The interactive objective takes into account that different abilities may be required for different trials. Grisso (1988) encourages experts to make a *conclusory* opinion or address the ultimate legal question in their evaluation, though he recognizes that other experts will disagree that such opinions should be offered and encourages individual experts to make the decision on their own. Finally, Grisso (1988) argues that the forensic psychologist should gather information that is relevant to the disposition of the defendant to offer *prescriptive* recommendations. Information that addresses the likelihood of the defendant responding to treatment and the best available programs will assist the court in determining the best option for a defendant. Even though the goal of the competency evaluation is not to determine whether the defendant needs treatment, addressing the best course of action to address any deficits does assist the court in adjudicating a defendant in the long run.

As previously noted, it is important to assess for malingering in any forensic evaluation and competence is no exception. Despite the low threshold for competency, the nature of the potential deficits (e.g., lack of understanding of legal concepts, unwillingness to communication with attorney) and the ability to delay a criminal conviction may encourage defendants awaiting trial to malinger. Currently, the degree to which defendants attempt to malinger on CST evaluations is not clear. Forensic psychologists have estimated that over 15% of their CST evaluations are colored by malingering (Rogers, Salekin, Sewell, Goldstein, & Leonard, 1998; Rogers, Sewell, & Goldstein, 1994). In one study, Gothard, Viglione, Meloy, and Sherman (1995) found that 12.7% competency referrals were malingered. Research has even suggested that many of the previously reviewed competency measures are at risk for individuals feigning or malingering mental illness (Rogers, Sewell, Grandjean, & Vitacco, 2002). However, one competency to stand trial measure, the Evaluation of Competency to Stand Trial – Revised (ECST-R), specifically assesses respondents' attempts to feign incompetency and has shown some success (Rogers, Jackson, Sewell, & Harrison, 2004; Rogers et al., 2002). Whether a specific measure such as the ECST-R is used or not, an evaluation of malingering is an important aspect to any competency evaluation.

Characteristics of incompetent defendants

By identifying the characteristics of those defendants who are found to be incompetent or competent, we obtain some insight into those characteristics more likely to lead to a particular legal decision and the clinical decision-making process of the experts in the field, given the extremely high rate of agreement between expert opinions and the final legal decision (Zapf et al., 2004). Nicholson and Kugler's (1991) review identified a number of variables related to decisions of competence and incompetence. Since that time, more recent studies have further identified these characteristics. Cochrane, Grisso, & Frederick (2001) examined 1,710 federal defendants and found that 43% of those receiving a psychotic diagnosis, 38% receiving an organic diagnosis and 30% receiving a diagnosis of mental retardation were found to be incompetent to stand trial. Another study found that defendants suffering from a psychotic disorder were five times more likely to be found incompetent (Zapf et al., 2004). A recent study continued this trend and also clearly found that although diagnoses such as psychosis were related to incompetence, the majority of psychotic defendants were found competent (Warren et al., 2006).

Concern has arisen since an early study of competency found that demographic variables (e.g., age, ethnicity) were better at predicting competency than clinical variables (e.g., current symptoms) (Rogers, Gillis, McMain, & Dickens, 1988). The concern arose because if demographic variables were key determiners of competency, it would be suggestive of bias. However, more recent research has not supported this early finding. Hart and Hare (1992) did not find any age or race bias and again identified psychosis as the biggest determiner of a finding of incompetence. Cooper and Zapf (2003) found that employment status was the only demographic variable that predicted incompetence in 468 criminal defendants awaiting trial and referred for competency evaluations. Moreover, employment status is probably a variable related to mental illness in that mentally ill individuals are less likely to be employed. A recent study though did find that, across 12 years and over 8,000 evaluations, older, minority defendants were more likely to be identified as incompetent, though other factors were more important in determining competency (Warren et al., 2006). At this time, it does not seem that a clear conclusion can be offered about the relationship between competency and demographic factors.

Although criminal charges are not a formal element in competency standards, many forensic psychologists encourage use of contextual elements in competency evaluations (Zapf et al., 2006). However, research has been inconsistent regarding contextual factors such as the alleged crime (see Warren et al., 2006). Nonetheless, even those studies that have found different rates of competence among defendants, depending on the severity of the charge, have found that the differences for crime severity disappear when controlling for other variables like mental illness (Cochrane et al., 2001; Cooper & Zapf, 2003). Even if defendants who commit more severe crimes are more likely to be found competent, these relationships are not as significant as the relationships for psychopathology in explaining final competency decisions (Warren et al., 2006). These results suggest that crime severity is related to mental illness and that mental illness is the variable that is actually related to a finding of competence or incompetence.

Other Variables Related to Competence

There are other variables related to findings of competence. Studies have examined professional differences between forensic psychologists and forensic psychiatrists in conducting competence evaluations. Forensic psychologists are more likely to use collateral information, produce more clinical notes, and complete reports that are rated as more useful by legal professionals (Petrella & Poythress, 1983). Even though forensic psychologists and psychiatrists do not differ in their view of the importance of psychological testing, forensic psychologists are much more likely to use psychological testing in competency evaluations than forensic psychiatrists (Borum & Grisso, 1995). Warren et al. (2006) found that psychologists conduct more and longer interviews with defendants, spend more time preparing the competency evaluations, and were more likely to use psychological and neuropsychological testing. These findings are especially interesting given that trial judges and attorneys favored psychiatrists over psychologists in conducting evaluations for the court (Redding, Floyd, & Hawk, 2001). Results also suggest that psychologists may be more likely to find defendants incompetent than psychiatrists (Warren et al., 2006).

Another aspect of the competency evaluation that has been examined is the setting in which the evaluation took place (Warren, Rosenfeld, Fitch, & Hawk, 1997). Historically, competence evaluations have taken place in inpatient settings such as a mental health hospital. However, these evaluations are increasingly taking place on an outpatient basis (Grisso, Cocozza, Steadman, Greer, & Fisher, 1996). Such changes are largely cost saving in nature but also may have important implications for the ultimate determination of competency. Although some research has not found any differences (Edens, Poythress, Nicholson, & Otto, 1999), other studies have found differences in competency evaluation across settings (Heilbrun & Collins, 1995; Warren et al., 1997, 2006). Heilbrun and Collins (1995) found that 47% of outpatient settings used psychological testing while only 13% of inpatient settings used psychological testing. Warren et al. (2006) found that evaluations in inpatient settings involved more evaluators and more frequent clinical interviews but overall took less time than outpatient evaluations. There also were differences in the collateral information requested and collected as well as the type of testing utilized.

Scope of Practice in Competency Evaluations

As in the previous chapters, it is important to examine the limitations of clinical practice in regard to competency evaluations. You may believe that because competency is the most frequently addressed mental health issue and the threshold for competency is low that there is little concern about the potential limitations. However, commentators have argued that there are numerous problems with competency evaluations (Bardwell & Arrigo, 2002). For example, Bardwell and Arrigo (2002) argue that mental health professionals sometimes confuse competency and insanity and perform evaluations that attempt to address both issues simultaneously while misapplying the standards of each to the other. Skeem, Golding, Cohn, and Berge (1998) found that in 100 randomly selected competence to stand trial evaluations, evaluators rarely incorporated legally relevant information or addressed the reasoning underlying their psycholegal conclusions.

Another concern is that because there is a high rate of agreement between mental health evaluations and judicial determinations of competency, a default legal decision is being made by the evaluating forensic psychologist. Winick (1995b) has commented that the courts have simply delegated their decision making capacity to mental health professionals and thereby obscured the differences between legal and clinical decisions. Agreement between opinions rendered by forensic psychologists and final judicial determinations are frequently estimated above 90%. One study only found a single departure in over 300 competency evaluations (Zapf et al., 2004). The 90% figure may be an underestimate because the competency process is frequently not completed because criminal charges are dropped or the cases are plea bargained. One study even reported that in a majority of cases (59%), judges failed to hold a formal hearing and simply relied on the competency reports provided by the mental health professionals to make an informal decision (Roesch & Golding, 1980). It could be argued that if the competency reports are being used as the sole basis for legal determination, a forensic psychologist is by extension addressing a legal question and not a psychological one anymore. However, it is not clear that the high rate of agreement is a result of the legal system abdicating its responsibility or is a reflection of the relatively low threshold for competency and the high quality of the reports.

Restoration of Competency

Even though treatment is not directly relevant to the issue of competency, treatment or restoration of competency is typically the major emphasis for those individuals judged incompetent. As we previously stated, *Jackson v. Indiana* (1972) concluded that incompetent defendants "cannot be held more than a reasonable period of time to determine whether there is substantial probability that [they] will attain capacity in the foreseeable future" (p. 738). Though treatment response is not an inherent part of competency decisions, jurisdictions often include provisions for a determination of competence restoration after a defendant has been found incompetent (Nicholson & McNulty, 1992). **Competency restoration** refers to the process by which an incompetent defendant's competency is restored so that the legal process can continue. The restoration of competency can be accomplished through the use of psychotropic medication, psychotherapy, and psychoeducational interventions in which the incompetent defendant is educated about the legal system. Competency restoration tends to be successful, as less than one-quarter of incompetent defendants are identified as unlikely to be restored to competence upon an initial evaluation (Warren et al., 2006) and less than 10% of incompetent defendants are ultimately unable to be restored to competency (Nicholson, Barnard, Robbins, & Hankins, 1994; Nicholson & McNulty, 1992).

In general, incompetent defendants face short hospitalizations. Nicholson & McNulty (1992) found that the average length of stay for 150 randomly selected incompetent defendants was 68.8 days and that only 5.5% of defendants were held for six months. However, most studies suggest that incompetent defendants are more likely to be hospitalized for 4 to 6 months (Bennett & Kish, 1990; Golding, Eaves, & Kowaz, 1989; Rodenhauser & Khamis, 1988). Although *Jackson* did not define a reasonable amount of time, these results appear to be in keeping with the Court's mandate. There were also several variables related to length of stay in the hospital. Older, Caucasian, unemployed, defendants with previous psychiatric admissions, who were living alone or in an institution, and were diagnosed with psychoses or an organic disorder experienced longer hospitalizations (Nicholson & McNulty, 1992).

The low base rate of defendants not restored to competency presents a problem for identifying the characteristics that are related to poor treatment response in incompetent defendants. Golding (1992b) has suggested that poor functioning prior to onset of a mental illness, negative symptoms (i.e., symptoms that are characterized by an omission of normal characteristics such as inappropriate or flatted affect), a quick onset of symptoms, past psychiatric history, and a history of treatment response are the best predictors of treatment response in incompetent defendants. Carbonell, Heilbrun, & Friedman (1992) attempted to identify a list of predictors in a sample of defendants originally judged incompetent and included 38% of the sample that were not restored to competency within 3 months. Although they were able to identify those individuals who could not be restored with an accuracy of 77.2% in the original sample, they were only able to reach 59.5% accuracy using those same variables on a follow-up sample with the same high base rate of incompetent defendants who were not restorable (38%).

Nonetheless, most studies do not have sufficient numbers of individuals who could not be restored to competency and instead examine variables related to predictions made by the evaluators as to restoration capability. Hubbard & Zapf (2003) examined the variables related to competency restoration in a small sample of incompetent defendants of which some were deemed restorable (37.1%), some unable to regain competency (21.3%), and some who did not have a prediction clearly identified on the original report (41.6%). They found that those individuals who were restored to competency were more likely to have a previous criminal history, a current violence charge, a minor non-psychotic diagnosis, previous mental health contact, previous hospitalization, and prior use of psychotropic medication. These results were similar to a larger sample from the same researchers (Hubbard, Zapf, & Ronan, 2003). Another study found that those individuals deemed uncertain or unlikely to be restorable were older and men. Unlikely restoration candidates also were less likely to have prior convictions and more likely to be diagnosed with psychotic and mood disorders (Warren et al., 2006). There may be some consensus in the limited research that defendants unlikely to be restored suffer from more severe mental illnesses and have less extensive criminal histories.

Competency Restoration Programs

There has been surprisingly little research on competency restoration and treatment of defendants found incompetent at a time when some have questioned the effectiveness of the treatment of incompetent defendants (Mumley, Tillbrook, & Grisso, 2003). The lack of research may be because competency restoration is simply the implementation of traditional treatment approaches to improve overall mental health but this notion seems counterintuitive in light of the increasing use of specialized forensic units to treat these types of offenders (Clark, Holden, Thompson, Watson, & Wightman, 1993). Unlike the movement of the evaluation process to outpatient sources, the treatment of incompetent defendants has largely remained within inpatient facilities (Miller, 2003). Research comparing the two approaches is even less available than empirical support of competency restoration in general.

An initial step in most competency restoration interventions is the administration of medication, primarily to reduce psychotic symptoms (Cooper & Grisso, 1997). This approach seems very relevant given the relationship between psychosis and an initial finding of incompetence and the restorability of incompetent defendants. Nicholson and Kugler (1991) conducted a meta-analysis and found that incompetent defendants were more likely to suffer from a psychotic diagnosis, exhibit severe mental illness, and have been previously hospitalized. The typical incompetent defendant exhibits significant psychiatric impairment and legal parties appear to take this impairment into account when referring individuals for competency evaluations. However, the administration of medication is not a routine matter when dealing with incompetent defendants. For some defendants, it may seem a very reasonable choice to refuse medication in order to avoid prosecution. However, the Court has continually upheld the state's right to forcibly medicate individuals (*Riggins v. Nevada*, 1992; *Sell v. United States, 2002; Washington v. Harper*, 1990). Not only do *Sell* and the other cases solidify the government's right to involuntarily medicate a defendant but research suggests that incompetent defendants do not routinely refuse medication for legal strategy but instead do so because of delusions about their medication or denial of their mental illness (Ladds & Convit, 1994).

In addition to medication, competency restoration typically involves an educational or psychoeducational component. When talking about competency restoration in my class, I typically go into an elaborate discussion about the complexity of the process and state that it is very difficult to try to communicate the precise nature of such an involved process to students. Then I flip on the videotape of a courtroom scene from the movie *Few Good Men* or an episode of the television show *Law & Order* (see Figure 8.1). I then whip out a hastily

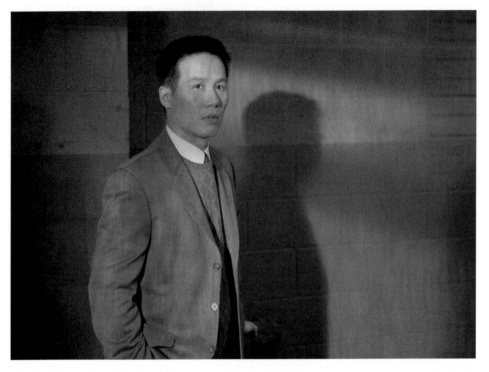

Figure 8.1. A picture of the fictional character, Dr. George Huang. *Law & Order* and B. D. Wong (Huang) have been publicly acknowledged for their accurate portrayal of forensic psychology/psychiatry. © Universal TV/The Kobal Collection

drawn picture of a courtroom with a judge's bench, a jury box, the two tables for the attorneys and the other respective participants and quiz the class about where everyone sits and their purpose. Obviously, my previous comments about the complexity of the process seem ridiculous because this aspect of competency restoration tends to be straight forward. Remember, the threshold for competency is very low. A defendant needs to be able to communicate with her attorney and understand the nature of the legal proceedings. If a defendant is medicated and her delusional belief that she is Britney Spears has been addressed, she may only need to be educated about the nature and consequences of the process. Can she identify the judge and jury? Are they out to get her or are they supposed to be objective and help decide whether she is ultimately guilty? These are the types of issues that are addressed in the psychoeducational component of competency restoration.

Generally, these types of approaches have been effective. Siegel and Elwork (1990) described a psychoeducational group that met for one hour each week for seven weeks. The group consisted of lectures, videotaped presentations, use of courtroom models, role-playing, and problem solving focused specifically on the competency to stand trial. A control group received identical treatment in terms of the length and time involved but it focused on more general mental health problems. Results showed that the experimental group in the specially designed treatment group showed greater improvement and were more likely to be recommended as competent.

However, there may be some issues in applying these findings to all incompetent defendants. It is not always the case that defendants found incompetent receive specialized treatment. Incompetent defendants often have received the same general treatment as civilly committed psychiatric patients (Grisso, 1992) and the general conditions in mental health hospitals have been criticized (Winick, 1983). Courts have even stated that incompetent defendants are often committed to maximum security wards at mental hospitals and this may be contrary to effective treatment (*Covington v. Harris*, 1969). Given these criticisms, it is important to realize that any traditional treatment for incompetent defendants is not necessarily going to be effective, but specialized psychoeducational treatment appears to be effective if patients are able to pay attention, concentrate, and cooperate (Brown, 1992). It also can be argued that some psychoeducational treatments encourage an artificial competence in that defendants, especially defendants suffering from mental retardation, may be able to pass a multiple choice exam on the different components of a courtroom because of their immediately recent education but not truly improve in their inherent understanding and assistance during the process. Furthermore, defendants receiving treatment involuntarily also benefit (Ladds & Convit, 1994); in fact, one study has shown that defendants who initially refused medication were more likely to be restored to competency (Rodenhauser & Khamis, 1988). Finally, there is very little information on incompetent defendants who are restored to competency and recidivism rates. Beckham, Annis, and Bein (1986) conducted a small study and found that 14% of patients who were restored to competency recidivated and that a decrease in medication at discharge and facing a more severe charge were related to recidivism.

Other Criminal Competencies

The discussion so far has focused on competency to stand trial because of the expansive literature on this aspect (Zapf et al., 2002) and the legal decisions equating different competency issues (*Godinez v. Moran*, 1993). Despite encouragement by the legal system to treat competency identically across different points in the adjudication process, scholars continue to argue for context specific competency evaluations in which the particular abilities necessary to plead, confess, be sentenced or be executed are examined. However, there are still other scholars that argue there is not empirical support for the notion that different contexts require different abilities, despite the calls in the literature to treat them as such (Coles, 2004).

Competency to Be Executed

Though the U.S. Supreme Court has ruled that two groups of defendants in which competency is a significant issue (i.e., those suffering from mental retardation and juveniles) are not eligible for the death penalty, competency for execution is raised with increasing frequency (Heilbrun, 1987). Prohibitions against executing an incompetent defendant have historical roots separate from general competency and can be traced back to the thirteenth-century notion that someone facing execution should be able to put his or her spiritual affairs in order to prepare to face God (Heilbrun, 1987). Competency to be executed may be a more frequent issue because of the stress experienced by those convicted and serving years on death row. In *Ford v. Wainwright* (1986), the U.S. Supreme Court case formally recognizing the competency rights of defendants facing execution, Alvin Ford began to show increasingly delusional behavior while on death row. His odd behavior began with the occasional peculiar idea but grew more serious and included a complex conspiracy involving the Ku Klux Klan and the prison guards, torture and abuse of his female relatives, a hostage crisis involving his family members, and his appointment as Pope. Though the Court recognized that Ford was not sufficiently competent to be executed, it did not identify a specific standard for competency to be executed. Nonetheless, research has begun to examine specialized forensic measures to be used in these evaluations (Ackerson, Brodsky, & Zapf, 2005; Zapf, Boccaccini, & Brodsky, 2002). Competency for Execution (CFE) evaluations may be especially problematic for forensic psychologists because of the inherent political and ethical issues involved in capital punishment. As a result, forensic psychologists must be aware of their personal biases when rendering these conclusions (see Chapter 3).

Competence to Waive Miranda Rights

Another area of competence that has received attention is the ability to confess and waive the right to counsel. In the United States, the ability to confess and waive counsel is tied to the Supreme Court decision *Miranda v. Arizona* (1966) in which specific criteria were identified for suspects to be interrogated and make confessions. As a result, competency to confess and competency to waive one's *Miranda* rights are often interchangeable in the United States (Brodsky & Bennett, 2005), even though there are other factors that should be considered in assessing whether a confession is valid (Greenfield & Witt, 2005). *Miranda* established that suspects must have the ability to knowingly, voluntarily, and intelligently waive their rights. Grisso (2003b) stated that a suspect must be able to understand the words and phrases included in the Miranda warning and be clear about the purpose of the Miranda warning, such as an awareness of the adversarial nature of the legal system and the right against self-incrimination. There have been specialized forensic measures developed to assess competency to confess but there is disagreement about the reliability and validity of those instruments (Grisso, 2004; Rogers, Jordan, & Harrison, 2004). On the other hand, competence to waive counsel was an issue in the trial of Colin Ferguson. Colin Ferguson went on a killing spree in December 1993 in which he killed 6 passengers on a New York commuter train and wounded 19 others. He continually insisted and was finally granted the right to serve as his own counsel and present his case to the jury. Even though he was able to object effectively to several aspects of the prosecutor's case, his unusual behavior and the suggestion that it was another man who opened fire on the train eventually led to him serving six consecutive life sentences.

Competency to Refuse the Insanity Defense

Another competency issue facing the courts is competence to refuse the insanity defense. Though the courts have not been completely consistent on the issue (Litwack, 2003), *Frendak v. United States* (1979) did find that a defendant must understand the plea's availability and the consequences of entering an insanity plea. The ability to refuse an insanity defense was a central feature in the criminal trial of Ted Kaczynski, the notorious Unabomber. Kaczynski mailed several bombs to numerous people who worked in university and industry settings over three decades because of a belief in the inherent evils of technological progress. His actions resulted in the death of 3 individuals and wounding of almost 30 others. Kaczynski was adamant at trial that he would not pursue a plea of insanity, against his attorneys' advice, because he did not want to be seen as mentally ill. He believed being mentally ill would diminish the credibility of his claims about technological progress. However, he agreed to a plea to avoid the death penalty and the issue was not decided by the court (Box 8.2).

Civil Competencies

Completely separate from the criminal competencies, are the civil aspects to competency. Competency is raised in a variety of issues including employment, professional competency, competency of a witness, competency to consent to sexual activity, competency to participate in mediation, competency to make a will, competency to enter into a contract, competency to make medical decisions. These areas are just a few of them. Civil competencies generally focus on an individual's ability to understand any of the information that is relevant to making an everyday decision. An individual must be able to understand the information relevant to the decision, apply that information to their situation, use rational thought to evaluate the benefits and consequences of any decision and communicate the decision (Grisso, 2003b). It could be argued that the specific threshold or standard for civil competency is more dependent on the context of the decision than the adjudicative competencies previously examined

Box 8.2. The Case for Competency with Ted Kaczynski

Ted Kaczynski was labeled the Unabomber after his almost two decade long string of mail bombings in the United States during the late 1970s and early 1990s. However, Kaczynski was not just some crazed lunatic acting without any awareness of the world around him. Ted Kaczynski was born and raised in Chicago and the school system recognized he was a bright child early on in his life. He was allowed to skip a grade and eventually graduated from high school and was admitted to Harvard University at age 16. After graduating from Harvard, he earned a PhD in mathematics from the University of Michigan and obtained an appointment in the mathematics department at the University of California-Berkeley. He soon resigned his position and began his series of bombings, starting with the first package addressed to a Northwestern professor in 1978 and ending with the murder of the head of the California Forestry Association in 1995. The rationale for his mail bombings was laid out in his 35,000 word paper titled, *Industrial Society and its Future*, or more commonly called the Unabomber's Manifesto in which he argued against the use of modern technology. Kaczynski's younger brother turned him into the FBI after he recognized aspects of the Manifesto. Kaczynski eventually plead guilty to avoid the death penalty and is serving a life sentence without the possibility of parole.

A significant issue in preparing for the trial was Kaczynski's refusal to plead insanity, despite his attorneys continued insistence. However, a defendant must be competent not only to stand trial but to also refuse an insanity defense. In examining his competency to stand trial and his aborted attempt at defending himself in court, there are several aspects which would support his competency. Kaczynski was extremely intelligent, understood the legal system, was able to communicate with his attorneys, understood the consequences of any verdict, and was socially skilled enough to deliver appropriate courtroom behavior in his defense. However, there were several characteristics that put his competency in question. He was diagnosed as suffering from paranoid schizophrenia and suffered from significant delusional beliefs outlined in his Manifesto. He had continued problems with authority figures, was uncooperative with his attorneys and would have been likely to have difficulty testifying and staying on track if he testified. Kaczynski's case is a reasonable example of the difficulty in assessing competency for many individuals who show clear strengths and clear deficits that may relate to their ability to understand legal proceedings and assist in their defense.

because of the greater variety of contexts in which an issue of civil competence may arise.

Competence to Treatment

Informed consent is typically required for any individual seeking medical care and usually consists of the health care professional identifying the risks and benefits. However, health care providers can act without consent if the patient is unable to give consent because of incapacitation, there is a greater risk of harm if treatment is delayed, a reasonable person would consent, or the person would normally consent to treatment (Slovenko, 2006). In some cases, a determination by the court must be made whether any of these conditions apply. For example, mentally ill individuals may be unable to make a treatment decision. Though research suggests that the majority of the mentally ill are competent to make treatment decisions, there are a number of mentally ill individuals who are not competent to make these decisions (Grisso & Appelbaum, 1995). Because these issues do not arise in the midst of legal proceedings, treatment decisions are often delayed or consent is sought from family or institutional boards. When these issues come before a court, there are instruments designed to assess competency relative to treatment with varying degrees of psychometric soundness. The MacArthur Competence Assessment Tool for Treatment (MacCAT-T) is one of the more recently developed measures (Grisso & Appelbaum, 1998) and is related to three other measures that were previously designed to assessment competence to make treatment decisions. The MacCAT-T consists of an interview focused on understanding the disorder, appreciation of the disorder, understanding treatment, understanding the risks and benefits of treatment, appreciation of treatment, awareness of alternative treatments, patient choice and the consequences of the choice (Grisso & Appelbaum, 1998). Competency to treat has undergone significant improvement in the past 20 years but there appears to be room for improvement in the development of measures and the application of these measures to the clinical evaluations.

Competence to Execute A Will

Every person who makes a will must be able to make competent decisions about the division of his or her property and personal belongings. The person making a will, the **testator**, must understand the nature of the property, identify the individuals eligible to receive the property upon death and the specific property to be assigned to them (Slovenko, 2006). Usually, the only way for a potential heir to contest or challenge a will is to challenge the capacity or competency of the testator to make the will. It should be clear that a testator does not have to be competent to formally write out the will, an attorney will do that part. He or she must have the capacity to make competent decisions about the division of the property. The threshold for competency to execute a will is relatively low compared to the competency to perform other civil responsibilities such as entering into a contract (Slovenko, 2006). In *Banks v. Goodfellow* (1870), the legal standards for competency to execute a will were established so that a person must know they are making a will, know the nature of the property, and know the manner in which the will distributed the property.

Performing competency evaluations for the execution of a will can be especially difficult. The person of interest is often dead and not available to be directly assessed. As a result, the evaluator must often rely on past records and information from third parties to assess the competency of the testator. Even though the threshold for competency to execute a will is low, the presence of a mental illness is not sufficient to find someone incompetent (Melton et al., 1997). These evaluations typically focus on the testators' functional abilities as they relate to the relevant legal criteria such as understanding the purpose of the will. The forensic psychologist also must determine the extent of the testator's property and the relationship between the testator and his or her family and friends that might suggest their preferences. These types of evaluations appear to be less structured with varying standards of practice than the previous areas, which might have had structured measures or interviews, developed for the specific purpose.

Competency Related to Guardianship

Guardianship is the identification of an individual by the state to make legal decisions for another person who is no longer able and may be the oldest issue in mental health law (Melton et al., 1997). All individuals are naturally assumed to be competent so a guardian is appointed after it has been determined in court that an individual is no longer able to make competent decisions in her own best interest. A guardian may be necessary for a variety of reasons. A person may be unable to make decisions in regard to her own health care, the use of her own financial resources, or caring for any of a person's basic needs. Moye (2003) believes that guardianship evaluations may be the most difficult in all of forensic psychology because of the broad issues that must be addressed in them.

Determining the need for guardian may be fairly easy if the person is civilly committed or otherwise incapacitated. Therefore, competency evaluations are more likely necessary when this situation has not arisen. In these instances, a person must petition the court to find someone incompetent and in need of a guardian. Though these decisions may be the most difficult for forensic psychologists, they tend to be the most informal from a legal standpoint (Melton et al., 1997). For example, many states do not require formal evaluations (Thor, 1993). As per other competency issues, clinicians should emphasize the functional abilities of the person as they relate to the specific task or even a broad range of tasks, if they are relevant to the question before the court. At least one measure has been developed for the assessment of guardianship, the Community Competence Scale (CCS). The CCS was developed to assess daily life skills across 16 different subscales in order to improve the reliability and validity of these types of evaluations (Searight, Oliver, & Grisso, 1983). There are also a variety of measures that focus on related abilities such as daily living skills, neuropsychological and cognitive deficits, and mental health problems (Moye, 2003). It is also important to the evaluator in these instances to identify whether any deficits are the result of incompetence or a lack of education or experience.

Summary

Competence related to criminal proceedings is often referred to as adjudicative competence and is based on the idea that in order to make criminal proceedings fair, a person must exhibit a basic ability to understand and participate in the process. Even though ensuring competence is meant to maintain the fairness of the process and is a mental health issue facing the legal system, it is separate from determinations of insanity. Competency focuses on a person's mental state at the present time whereas insanity refers to specifically a person's mental state at the time of the alleged crime. Insanity is also a legal defense to a criminal charge and while competency may delay a trial it is not a defense that would acquit a defendant of criminal wrongdoing. There are also different standards or thresholds for competency compared to insanity that suggest the threshold to be found incompetent is much higher than for a defendant to be found insane.

Competency to Stand Trial (CST) is probably the most prevalent mental health issue addressed by the legal system with competency evaluations occurring in between 2% and 8% of all felony cases. Questions about the competence of a defendant may be raised at anytime by the judge or any of the attorneys and may result in a formal evaluation being conducted by a forensic psychologist. After the evaluation has been completed the parties may stipulate to the competence of the defendant or the judge may make a final determination. If a defendant is found incompetent to stand trial there is a delay in the trial until the defendant is either restored to competency or the charges dropped.

There is not a single approach for conducting a competency evaluation and therefore there is significant variability among forensic psychologists. Competency evaluations may consist of traditional psychological tests designed to assess cognitive and psychological abilities and specialized forensic instruments designed to assess competency to stand trial. A number of these specialized competence instruments have been developed and are currently in use. In addition to these instruments, a model for competency evaluations has been suggested that emphasizes functional, causal, interactive, conclusory, and prescriptive dimensions.

There tends to be a low threshold for finding someone competent and incompetent defendants tend to be significantly impaired. Incompetent defendants are likely to suffer from psychosis and there may be typical demographic and criminal history variables associated with them. There also are certain characteristics associated with competency evaluations. Studies have generally found that there are differences in evaluations depending on whether they have been conducted by forensic psychologists or psychiatrists, the setting that the evaluation has taken place in, and the methods employed.

Another issue involved in competency is the restoration of competency. Competency restoration is necessary when a defendant has been deemed incompetent and the legal proceeding is delayed as a result. A defendant's competency may be restored via standard psychological interventions such as the administration of medication or the use of psychotherapy. There also are specialized programs that have been devised that focus on psychoeducational aspects of competency restoration and have proven to be effective. As with other aspects of forensic practice, there also are scope of practice issues related to competency determinations.

In addition to competency to stand trial there are other related criminal competencies and civil competencies. Other areas of criminal competence include the need for individuals to be competent when facing execution, waiving their rights to confess or obtain counsel (Miranda rights in the United States), and refuse the insanity defense. Civil competencies are similar to criminal competencies in that they focus on an individual's ability to make decisions. However, they are dissimilar in that they are less likely to involve formal legal hearings and focus on a broader range of contexts and abilities. Common civil issues may be competence to make treatment decisions, execute a will, or appoint a guardian.

Key Terms

competency restoration   functional abilities   testator
fitness   in absentia

Further Reading

Grisso, T. (2003a). *Evaluating competencies: Forensic assessments and instruments*. New York: Kluwer Academic/Plenum Publishers.

9 Civil Commitment

Another issue related to competency and insanity is the civil commitment or involuntary hospitalization of the mentally ill. Though civil commitment is distinct from insanity and competency, it is also related to these two other aspects of mental health law. Competence to give informed consent or competence to refuse medical treatment (see Chapter 8) have direct application to civil commitment because these individuals are frequently civilly committed in order to treat their mental health issues. Individuals who have been found NGRI are routinely civilly committed immediately after their acquittal. However, there are also clear differences between competency, insanity, and civil commitment. Despite the significant legal and practice differences between insanity, competency, and civil commitment, it is easy to get them confused. First, although they focus on someone's mental state, insanity and civil commitment both explicitly require the presence of a mental disorder or defect, while competency does not in many jurisdictions. Second, competency tends to focus on someone's present mental state, insanity focuses on past mental state, and civil commitment focuses both on present and future mental state because it may require an assessment of future dangerousness. Third, insanity is raised in criminal proceedings, civil commitment is a civil issue, and competency can be either a criminal or civil issue (see Table 9.1).

In particular, civil commitment was not established to ensure fairness in the criminal system, it was intended to assist individuals who suffered from mental illness and were in need of treatment. Nonetheless, the original intent of civil commitment has changed, especially in the United States, over the past several decades. The current chapter will focus on a number of different aspects of civil commitment including the elements that define it, the legal theory that guides it, and the clinical process involved.

Table 9.1.   Comparison of Civil Commitment, Insanity, and Competency

Civil commitment	Insanity	Competency
Requires presence of mental illness	Requires presence of mental illness	Does not require presence of mental illness
Focuses on future and present	Focuses on past	Focuses on present
Civil issue	Criminal issue	Civil and criminal issue

What is Civil Commitment?

Civil commitment typically refers to the involuntary hospitalization or mandated treatment of mentally ill individuals who need care and incapacitation because they exhibit dangerous tendencies toward themselves or others. The legal basis for civil commitment is usually described as originating out of the legal doctrine **parens patriae** or parent of the country. Under this theory, the state is obligated to act in a parenting capacity for those individuals who are unable to care for themselves. Accordingly, parens patriae is used as a basis for a number of legal provisions that involve minors, the mentally ill and the elderly. As parens patriae relates to the mentally ill, it suggests that the state not only has a right but a duty to protect people who may be at risk to themselves because they suffer from a mental illness. It emphasizes mental illness or an inability to care for oneself. A contrasting but related legal doctrine is **police power**. Under police power, the state's prominent obligation is not to protect the individual from himself but to protect society from that individual. The highest duty would be to protect society from any danger that may put the general citizenry at risk. Police power normally emphasizes dangerousness to others and therefore places a premium on prediction of dangerousness instead of an inability to care for oneself.

These two legal doctrines have shaped the development of civil commitment legislation and practice since its inception, thereby contributing to the therapeutic and anti-therapeutic consequences. Parens patriae served as a foundation for civil commitment laws prior to the latter half of the twentieth century. At the same time, civil commitment laws were largely based on a medical model that suggested the mentally ill could and should be treated for their disorders. Historically, the mentally ill were placed in mental health institutions for extended periods of time, if not the rest of their lives, at the discretion of mental health professionals. The basis for civil commitment under the notion of parens patriae was that the mentally ill were in need of treatment. Thus, it was in their best interest to allow the state to commit them to a facility where they could receive the proper treatment. In practice, these commitments generally only required the signature of one or two mental health professionals and did not even require the diagnosis of a precise mental illness or the presence of any dangerous tendencies. Parens patriae served as the

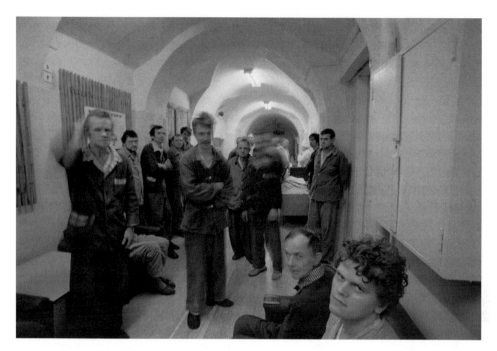

Figure 9.1.   A psychiatric hospital in Russia. © Bernard Bisson / Sygma / Corbis

theoretical basis for civil commitment until the 1960s. At this time, concern arose about the abuse of civil commitment and the realization that the institutionalization of citizens deprived them of significant rights. Mental health professionals lost their largely unchecked ability to civilly commit patients and the process became less entrenched in a medical model and more in line with legalistic notions. The 1960s were also marked by the widespread use of antipsychotic medications that allowed for the release of individuals who previously had been institutionalized their entire lives. Figure 9.1 shows a psychiatric hospital in Russia.

The 1960s and 1970s were characterized by a number of U.S. court cases in which limitations were placed upon the commitment process. For example, a federal court ruled in *Lake v. Cameron* (1966) that less restrictive alternatives should be considered instead of institutionalization and the widespread use of medication made less restrictive alternatives more likely. In another case, *Lessard v. Schmidt* (1972), individuals facing commitment were afforded a number of procedural safeguards for their liberty such as notice of the impending civil commitment procedures, the opportunity to state their case, and the right to representation. Cases like these and the Supreme Court cases that followed them, represented attempts to protect individuals facing potential commitments and marked the end of the states' unchecked institutionalization of anyone who exhibited unusual behavior. Recognition that civil commitment involved a significant loss of liberty (*Humphrey v. Cady*, 1972) and that

Box 9.1.   *O'Connor v. Donaldson* and the Case for Dangerousness

O'Connor v. Donaldson was an important case in mental health law, for civil commitment and even in the development of risk assessment. Kenneth Donaldson was a married man with three children prior to his significant mental health problems. His first difficulties began in his early 30s for which he was hospitalized and received electroconvulsive shock treatment. Upon release, he returned to living with his family until approximately a decade later. His second hospitalization occurred after he traveled to his parents' home in Florida and complained of paranoid delusions that he was being poisoned. His parents began commitment proceedings and he was soon committed to Chattahoochee State Hospital where he resided with dangerous criminals during his 15 year stay, even though he was never found to be a danger to himself or others. Donaldson further denied he was ever mentally ill during his stay at Chattahoochee and refused all treatment. He requested release on multiple occasions and even secured shelter and supervision if he was granted a release.

As a result of the hospital's continued refusal to release him, the American Civil Liberties Union (ACLU) took up Donaldson's case and argued that he had been deprived of his constitutional right to liberty because he was detained against his will and without treatment. The United States Supreme Court unanimously agreed and stated that a non-dangerous person who is able to survive on the outside on his own or with the assistance of others should be released. Though this case was one in a series that helped bolster support for the mentally ill and was intended to fight some of the abuses present in the mental health system, one of the important implications for civil commitment was the Court's conclusion that a mental illness alone was not sufficient for the indefinite commitment of an individual. One interesting aspect of the case is that Donaldson was actually released prior to his case ever being heard by the Court and immediately obtained a job. He lived on his own for years before his case was heard by the Supreme Court in 1975.

safeguards must be in place because of this recognition generally colored future Court decisions. In *O'Connor v. Donaldson* (1975), the United States Supreme Court concluded that a person not only had to be mentally ill but also dangerous before he could be civilly committed (see Box 9.1) and thereby encouraged significant scope of practice issues at the time, given the lack of research supporting risk assessment in any context. The intent of these legal changes was to reduce the number of people hospitalized. Evidence gathered since the widespread use of psychotropic medication and these legal decisions seem to suggest the intended effect. The number of people committed to public hospitals decreased from 1955 to 1965 from 558,000 to 475,000 (Kiesler & Simpkins, 1993) and was 132,000 as early as 1980 (Brakel, Parry, & Weiner, 1985). These additional protections also seemed to signal a swing from parens patriae to police power. The focus has moved away from the presence of a mental

Table 9.2.   Important Case Law in Civil Commitment

Case	Result
Lake v. Cameron (1966)	Required that treatment should be in the least restrictive setting
Lessard v. Schmidt (1972)	Commitment proceedings must include the same procedural safeguards as criminal proceedings such as a notice of the impending civil commitment procedures and the right to counsel
Wyatt v. Stickney (1972)	Established the right to receive treatment for individuals civilly committed with a realistic chance of improvement
O'Connor v. Donaldson (1975)	An individual must exhibit dangerousness in order to be civilly committed
Addington v. Texas (1979)	The standard of proof in civil commitment proceedings is clear and convincing evidence
Zinermon v. Burch (1990)	Mentally ill individuals are not able to give consent for voluntary admission

illness and the informal authority of mental health professionals toward the more legalistic focus of dangerousness. A number of formal procedures were designed to protect the person facing civil commitment as a result. Table 9.2 summarizes some important case law in civil commitment.

These changes have led to concerns that the mentally ill would be criminalized and concerns about the therapeutic impact of the law and related legal proceedings (see Chapter 2). These fears may have been realized as civilly committed individuals have increasingly had prior criminal justice involvement (Lamb & Grant, 1982). Evidence also suggests that alternative criminal mechanisms are used to divert individuals away from civil procedures. Some mentally ill individuals are arrested for minor crimes that normally would be dismissed and instead recommended for pretrial competency evaluations (Appelbaum, Fisher, Nestelbaum, & Bateman, 1992). Furthermore, a majority of judges in at least one jurisdiction have admitted they refer people who appear mentally ill for competency evaluations to ensure appropriate treatment (Appelbaum & Fisher, 1997). Although these actions may be well intended, there are serious concerns about using the criminal justice system in a potentially abusive manner to maneuver around legal safeguards.

Criteria for Civil Commitment

Similar to insanity and competency, there are specific criteria that are routinely found in civil commitment statutes. In order to be civilly committed a person must be mentally ill and dangerous. Although some states include additional criteria, the presence of a mental illness and the likelihood of future dangerousness represent universal criteria for commitment. However, there are several nuances to both of these criteria in the practice of civil commitment.

Mental Illness

The more prominent and long standing of the two criteria is the presence of a mental illness. However, there are several potential problems that immediately arise with a seemingly straightforward criterion. One question is whether the legal or medical bases for a mental disorder are used for civil commitment decisions. Is there a difference between the legal definition of mental illness and the medical or mental health definition? Practically speaking, there is a difference between the two with the legal definition of mental illness being narrower. Typically, when the term mental illness is used, mental health professionals identify disorders that are commonly found in the DSM. This practice leads to an inclusive list and encompasses almost every construct that is generally accepted by the mental health field as constituting a mental illness. However, the law generally picks and chooses mental illnesses it views as appropriate for a particular legal determination and is ambiguous about defining mental illness (*Foucha v. Louisiana*, 1992). Civil commitment is no different. Mental disorders such as mental retardation, substance abuse and dependence, antisocial personality disorder and even all personality disorders are routinely excluded from consideration as insufficient to meet this criterion under civil commitment statutes. These mental illnesses may be excluded from the legal definition of mental illness because they are chronic, believed to lack effective treatment, are perceived as a matter of personal choice and control, or are intertwined with antisocial or dangerous behavior that is characteristic of the second criterion for civil commitment. The reason for exclusion does not necessarily matter to the practicing forensic psychologist though, as long as she realizes there are legal limitations to the mental illnesses considered for civil commitment.

Another potential problem with the use of mental illness as a criterion for civil commitment is the seriousness of the mental illness. For example, personality disorders may be excluded from the legal definition of mental illness because they are seen as less severe or because they impair an individual to a lesser extent than other mental illnesses. Some statutes give no indication of the severity or level of impairment necessary for the civil commitment of an individual. Other statutes state that the mental illness has to impair someone to such an extent that he is unable to make decisions. Nonetheless, mental illnesses will impair an individual to a varying extent and the civil commitment laws seem to suggest this aspect is part of the definition of mental illness.

Another potential problem with mental illness is the presence of the hindsight bias. Who is more likely to be seen as mentally ill, a person who is not currently institutionalized and has never been institutionalized or someone who is hospitalized or even being evaluated for hospitalization? Rosenhan's (1973) famous experiment may give us the answer to that question (Box 9.2). One of

Box 9.2.   Rosenhan's Study: Insane in Insane Places

David Rosenhan published the results of his famous experiment in the journal *Science* in 1972. Rosenhan's study involved a series of associates acting as pseudopatients attempting to gain admission to 12 different psychiatric facilities in multiple locations across the United States. His associates presented themselves to hospital staff with a single fake symptom that consisted of an auditory hallucination. All of them claimed to hear a voice that was unclear but seemed to be saying words like empty and thud. They did not claim any other symptoms and all other information they reported was correct, except for their names and employment information. If admitted, they were to act normally and report they no longer heard the voices. All of them were eventually admitted, diagnosed with a major mental illness (seven with schizophrenia and one with bipolar disorder) and held anywhere from a week to almost two months. An interesting side note was that the patients in these very same facilities tended to be the ones who questioned whether the pseudopatients were faking their symptoms.

The publication of his research caused a great deal of discussion about its methods and the claim that it was an indictment of psychiatry in general. There also was a second part of the experiment that is often overlooked. Rosenhan repeated his experiment at a well regarded hospital that had heard of the results and did not believe the same outcome would occur at their facility. The hospital agreed to allow Rosenhan to send pseudopatients to them over a three month period. During that time the hospital reviewed 193 patients and identified 41 of them as suspected imposters by at least one staff member (attendants, nurses, physicians, or psychologists), 23 by one psychiatrist, and 19 by one psychiatrist and one other staff member. However, Rosenhan had never sent any pseudopatients to the hospital.

the lessons from this experiment was that there was a certain hindsight bias or labeling effect of anyone whose mental health might be questioned or institutionalized. When these patients presented themselves and certainly once they were admitted, there was a natural tendency for staff to view them in a way that was consistent with their hospitalization and their diagnosis.

Dangerousness

The second universal criterion for civil commitment is dangerousness, either a danger to self or a danger to others. As with mental illness, there is variability in the conceptualization of the nature of dangerousness. In terms of danger to others, most jurisdictions consider bodily harm to be the threshold requirement. However, some states suggest that danger to others could include property, other interests or even emotional harm. Some jurisdictions even require an overt act for danger to others to have been met. In terms of danger to self, statutes are even more vague and may or may not equate danger to self as suicidal attempts, gestures or ideation. Some jurisdictions use the term imminent risk of suicide but still frequently leave imminent undefined.

Much like with the mental illness criterion, problems also arise in addressing the dangerousness criterion for mental illness. As was discussed in Chapter 5, mental health professionals have historically had a great deal of difficulty predicting or assessing violence risk. This exercise has been especially problematic in committed psychiatric patients in part because of the controversy over the relationship of mental illness and violence. The literature has not always been clear about this relationship and inaccurate stereotypes of the mentally ill has made the communication of the available information even more difficult when relationships were found. The relationship between mental illness and violence will be discussed in more depth later in the chapter. Nonetheless, assessing risk is still difficult among civil psychiatric patients.

A second reason the assessment of risk is difficult is because of the use of actuarial and clinical approaches. Though an argument can be made for the superiority of actuarial approaches over clinical assessments of risk (Quinsey, Rice, Harris, & Cormier, 2006), the use of actuarial approaches is difficult when civil commitment decisions are necessary (Elbogen, Huss, Tomkins, & Scalora, 2005; Elbogen, Williams, Kim, Tomkins, & Scalora, 2001). Often these situations require fairly immediate decisions if an individual is presented for admission to a mental health facility or hospital emergency room. The individual may be uncooperative, records unavailable, and historical information generally difficult to obtain. As a result of the need for immediate decisions, clinical predictions are often the norm and therefore forensic psychologists are left with an approach that may be less accurate.

Related to the dangerousness to self requirement is the term **grave disability**. Most jurisdictions explicitly consider the presence of a grave disability to be sufficient for danger to self and all jurisdictions permit it. Someone is normally considered gravely disabled if they are unable to care for themselves and provide for their own basic needs. It is interesting that grave disability is the most frequent reason for civil commitment over dangerousness and that young persons (21–35) are the ones, not the elderly, who are typically committed on the basis of a grave disability (Turkheimer & Parry, 1992). One reason that mental health professionals may be more comfortable with a designation of grave disability is that it requires proof of a current deficit in one's ability to care for oneself, not a future or predicted inability (Wexler & Winick, 1991).

Need for Treatment

Another criterion for civil commitment that is not as universal as the presence of mental illness and dangerousness is the need for treatment. Although the need for treatment was the original basis for civil commitment, it is not sufficient in itself to support taking away an individual's liberty. The only other instance where the state is able to deprive citizens of liberty is when an

results. All participants were individuals who had been previously involuntarily committed as inpatients and were either released as outpatient commits or released without that supervision. Outpatient commitment did not result in reduced utilization of hospital services but participants who received extended outpatient commitments had fewer readmissions and fewer days in the hospital, if they were readmitted (Swartz et al., 1999). Furthermore, a combination of extended outpatient services and frequent utilization of services did relate to a reduction in overall violence (Swanson et al., 2000). Quality of life is another indicator of treatment success, though a more abstract one. The utilization of outpatient commitment is not only related to hospital readmission and criminal justice outcomes but is also related to improvement in general quality of life. Patients who underwent longer periods of outpatient commitment generally reported a greater quality of life (Swanson, Swartz, Elbogen, Wagner, & Burns, 2003a).

Coercion of Civil Commitments

Estimates have generally suggested that upwards of 30% of all psychiatric patients are involuntary committed (Monahan & Shah, 1989) but even among the remaining 70% of individuals, most are not truly voluntary. For example, individuals classified as voluntary may have been hospitalized under threat of a formal civil commitment. A U.S. Supreme Court decision further complicates the distinction between voluntary and involuntary admission. In *Zinermon v. Burch* (1990), the court ruled that individuals who are seriously mentally ill are not able to consent to a voluntary admission and therefore must be involuntarily committed. Research also has shown that though legal status (voluntary versus involuntary) is related to perception of coercion, there are important differences between being involuntarily committed and feeling coerced (Hiday, Swartz, Swanson, & Wagner, 1997; Hoge et al., 1997; Nicholson, Ekenstam, & Norwood, 1996). As a result, research has begun to ignore the distinction between voluntary and involuntary and focus more on the level of **coercion** the patient experiences or perceives they experience.

Coercion can mean the use of threats or force, medicating a patient against her will, or having police bring a patient to the hospital. Though there may not be a precise definition of coercion, there are several dimensions that have been taken into account (Wertheimer, 1993). These dimensions include the perceived availability of alternatives, strength of patient preferences for pursuing hospitalization versus alternatives, the type and intensity of the pressure placed on the patient, and the burden of choosing hospitalization. Moreover, coercion should be related to the context in which the behavior occurs because what may be coercive in one context is not coercive in another (Wertheimer, 1993). Though coercion is an inherent part of civil commitment, there has been debate about the level of coercion that is appropriate and the true nature of coercion (Lidz, 1998).

The Impact of Coercion on Civil Commitment

One fear is that undue coercion will lead to poor therapeutic relationships between clinicians and patients and thereby treatment effectiveness will be reduced and readmissions increased. Others suggest that many patients may only be thankful for care because they were coerced (Gardner & Lidz, 2001). However, 81% of clinicians believed that mandated community outpatient treatment deters people with schizophrenia from seeking voluntary treatment and 78% believed that legal pressures encouraged patients to stay in treatment. Furthermore, 36% of patients admitted that fear of coercive treatment reduced their chances of seeking mental health assistance and fear of coerced treatment was correlated with concerns about seeking treatment (Swartz, Swanson, & Hannon, 2003). Results suggest that coercive treatment is a barrier to patients seeking treatment and that clinicians may minimize the relationship between coercion and seeking treatment.

Until recently, there has been little research examining the role of coercion in civil commitment decisions. This literature has largely focused on reducing any potential harm to the patient by eliminating or reducing the perception that the civil commitment process is coercive (McKenna, Simpson, & Coverdale, 2000). For example Huss and Zeiss (2005) examined whether or not more fully explaining to patients that they had the right to a commitment hearing as well as the right to avoid a commitment hearing, reduced direct and indirect procedural indicators of coercion. These results were largely supportive of a reduction in coercion and better treatment outcome. Initially, efforts were aimed at defining and assessing coercions among psychiatric patients (Bennett et al., 1993, Gardner et al., 1993. Hoge et al., 1993). Though coercion has been measured in different ways, a standardized interview and measure do exist. The MacArthur Admission Experience Interview and the MacArthur Admission Experience Survey (Gardner et al., 1993) and several coercion-related behaviors have routinely been used: persuasion, inducement, threat, show of force, physical force, legal force, asked for a dispositional preference, giving an order, and deception (Lidz et al., 1997).

One question in the literature is whether patients change their original attitudes toward hospitalization during the hospitalization. Some have justified inpatient commitment on the theory that many patients change their mind about being hospitalized and are eventually grateful after receiving treatment. Gardner et al. (1999) interviewed 433 admitted patients at two different psychiatric hospitals. Results showed that the majority of patients believed they needed to be hospitalized (76%) and that over half (52%) of the patients who originally denied needing hospitalization later changed their minds. Patients who changed their minds did not differ from those who did not change their minds according to race, sex, age, anger about being hospitalized upon admission or severity of mental illness. However, change was related to believing one had a mental illness. Patients who believed they had a mental illness upon admission were more likely to change their mind.

Sources and Frequency of Coercion

Studies also have examined the sources of coercive behaviors among patients. One study found that mental health professionals were the most important source of coercion and that they exhibit several different types of coercion (Lidz et al., 2000). In fact, "it is the clinical pressures, not the behaviors of relatives, friends, or law enforcement personnel, that appear to account for patients' perceptions that they have been coerced" (p. 79). Furthermore, though patients, staff, and family/friends may share a common conceptualization of coercion in the admission process, patients' perceptions do not necessarily match staff perceptions of coercion (Hoge et al., 1998). Family members were less likely to report coercion and negative pressures related to the admission process (Hoge et al., 1998). Clinicians and patients also disagree on the level of coercion involved in issues such as forced medication, the involuntary nature of earlier commitments, and current legal status (Poulsen & Engberg, 2001). In general, there appears to be a "grey zone" (p. 60) between what patients' and clinicians' believe is coercive (Poulsen & Engberg, 2001). Patients' overall level of coercion is tied to a perception of the **procedural justice** involved in a situation. Procedural justice refers to the notion that an individual has been treated fairly in a given context, regardless of the outcome (Tyler, 2006). Patients who feel like they are not listened to or given a role in the process tend to report higher levels of coercion (Lidz et al., 1995) whereas clinicians' and family members' perceptions of coercion are not strongly related to issues involving procedural justice (Hoge, Lidz, et al., 1997; as cited in Lidz et al., 1997). In addition, further research has found that at times race (African–Americans felt less coerced), factors related to negative symbolic pressure (e.g., threats, giving orders, deception, show of force), and force (legal and physical force) are related to perceived coercion in commitment patients. Additional analyses did not find race consistently related to coercion though (Lidz et al., 1998).

The problem with much of the coercion research has been that it relies on patient reports. Patient reports can be potentially fallible both because of their position in the process and that their mental health issues may skew their perspective. Reports attempting a more comprehensive examination have found that there is not a single source of data that is completely adequate, though patient reports appear to be the most accurate (Lidz et al., 1997). The one exception to this finding was in regard to the use of force in which clinicians appear to be the most accurate sources of information. Moreover, the discrepancy between patient reports of coercion and other sources does not appear to be related to mental illness or severity of mental illness on a consistent basis (Lidz et al., 1997).

One question remains, how frequent is coercion? In general, persuasion is the most common method of coercion occurring in 61.6% of patients. The only other aspect of coercion that occurs in a majority of commitment patients was whether anyone asked about the patient's preference for hospital admission (56.8%), followed by legal force (33.1%), giving orders (28.5%), show of force

(22.8%), threats (18.6%), inducement (8.8%), deception (6.4%), and physical force (5.8%) (Lidz et al., 1998). Other research has found that while 70% of psychiatric patients believe their admissions were necessary, 74% felt they were under pressure to be hospitalized (Bonsack & Borgeat, 2005).

One way to prevent coercion is by following admission criteria and not allowing outside biases to enter the decision process. A positive finding along those lines is that clinicians appear to only rely on the commitment criteria (mental illness, dangerousness, and need for treatment) to retain individuals for civil commitment (Segal, Laurie, & Segal, 2001). Other factors such as the difficulty of the setting, patient's lack of insurance, patient's involuntary admission status, patient's level of participation in evaluation process, gender, and race do not relate to retention for civil commitment. However, the greater the workload experienced by the evaluating clinician, the more likely they are to retain a patient (Segal et al., 2001).

Right to Make Treatment Decision and Refuse Treatment

Another issue related to coercion during the commitment process is the right to make treatment-related decisions and refuse treatment. It has been argued that one way to make the treatment process less coercive is to involve patients in the treatment decision process. It is clear that individuals who have been civilly committed have a right to receive treatment. In *Wyatt v. Stickney* (1972), an Alabama law allowed for the commitment of individuals for "safe keeping." Originally, the plaintiffs sued the state of Alabama over cutbacks at the state mental hospital because of a budget shortfall. The plaintiffs happened to include Ricky Wyatt, a 15 year-old relative of a former employee at the Bryce State Mental Hospital, as a plaintiff. Though the Alabama courts ruled the state had a right to lay off staff, additional consideration was given to the treatment of Ricky Wyatt. Wyatt had been institutionalized, despite the lack of a mental illness, simply because he was identified as a juvenile delinquent. The suit charged that the conditions were horrible and treatment was only used to manage the behavior of the patients. Ultimately, the courts determined patients had a right to treatment that would give them a realistic opportunity to improve their mental condition. Although the right to treatment was limited in later decisions (*O'Connor v. Donaldson*, 1975; *Youngberg v. Romeo*, 1982), patients who have been involuntarily committed have basic rights regarding treatment.

The United States Supreme Court also addressed the right to refuse treatment on several occasions. On each occasion the Court recognized the right to refuse treatment but also recognized that the state often has legitimate interests in forced treatment. *Sell v. United States* (2003) held that a defendant who was hospitalized after being found incompetent to stand trial may be involuntarily medicated in some circumstances. Charles Sell was a practicing dentist with an

10

Domestic Violence and Stalking

As domestic violence cases increasingly enter the court system (Roehl & Guertin, 1998), forensic psychologists are correspondingly being asked to assist the courts. Forensic psychologists are performing several roles in domestic violence cases and are specifically being asked to:

> (1) describe the nature, frequency, severity, and consequences of previous violence; (2) make predictions about the likelihood and severity of future violence; (3) provide intervention recommendations for the batterer as well as for the victim; and (4) make predictions regarding the likely outcomes of these interventions. (Levensky & Fruzzetti, 2003, p. 713)

This chapter will focus on these specific aspects of domestic violence, which are very much in keeping with assessment and treatment in forensic psychology in general. However, domestic violence presents numerous challenges to forensic psychologists working in the area.

Before we begin, there are a couple of important issues to clarify. Most of the research in domestic violence has focused on male perpetrated domestic violence and this chapter will be no different. However, the research examining women as perpetrators of domestic violence and some of the potential differences in male perpetrated domestic violence will be considered, along with some of the societal implications. The ways in which the law plays a role in the practice of forensic psychology and the mental health of those involved is profound in domestic violence. Therapeutic jurisprudence is evident not only near the disposition and trial stage, as has been the case for much of our discussion so far, but also in the arrest or initial reporting of domestic violence. In addition, we will discuss a topic that is related to domestic violence, stalking. Though we know relatively little about stalking in comparison to domestic violence, the area has significantly expanded in terms of clinical practice and research over the past decade.

Defining and Identifying the Prevalence of Domestic Violence

As it was with risk assessment and general violence, it is important to define the nature of domestic violence. Domestic violence can mean any violence or aggression perpetrated within the context of a significant interpersonal relationship (e.g., family, marriage, dating). Domestic violence could include violence between a husband and a wife, a girlfriend and boyfriend, or gay and lesbian partners. It could include violence between parents and children (see Chapter 12 for a discussion of child abuse), between adult children and elderly parents, or even between siblings. However, this chapter will focus on domestic violence that occurs between men and women in an intimate partner relationship.

More specifically, domestic violence encompasses psychological, physical, and sexual aggression between intimate partners. One of the most prevalent measures used to assess domestic violence is the Conflict Tactics Scale (CTS). Students should be familiar with this somewhat controversial measure because it has become intertwined with the commonly accepted definitions of domestic violence and is central to understanding some of the issues involved in describing and estimating the prevalence of domestic violence. The revised version of the CTS, the Conflicts Tactics Scale-2 (CTS2), consists of items that offer examples of different aggressive behaviors that routinely occur in domestic conflicts (Straus, Hamby, Boney-McCoy, & Sugarman, 1996). These items can be further divided into the three broad categories of domestic violence (Table 10.1) and even physical aggression can be categorized into mild or moderate (e.g., arm twisting and hair pulling) and severe (e.g., using a knife or throwing an object that could hurt).

Factors that Influence Prevalence Figures

As a partial result of the definition and way in which we measure domestic violence there are not definitive prevalence rates. Some estimates suggest that as many as one-third of all women are victims of domestic violence during their lifetime (Straus & Gelles, 1990) and that four million women each year are assaulted by a domestic partner (see Sartin, Hansen, & Huss, 2006). However, these statistics should be examined cautiously in terms of their purpose and definitions of domestic violence. Did they include psychological aggression? Were the studies assessing members of the community or a high risk group of people? Are they estimates or more precise numbers arrived at through empirical research? For example, one review stated that as many as 57% of high school students and 65% of college students have been involved in violent relationships (Feldbau-Kohn, Schumacher, & O'Leary, 2000). However, these statistics include involvement both as a perpetrator and a victim of violence and include lifetime prevalence. Alternatively, many studies, especially those using the CTS or CTS2, only include violence occurring in the last year. Moreover, some forms of violence previously discussed, the victim may be repeatedly available to the perpetrator, increasing the opportunity for victimization. Should the punishment of the perpetrator be based on the continued presence of the victim? The issue of risk management becomes extremely important because of victim availability. As we will discuss, there are a variety of dynamic risk factors that can influence the perpetration of domestic violence and with the easier access to victims, identification of those factors and designing interventions specifically to reduce them or their impact is extremely important.

Because of the continued presence of the victim, many experts also encourage consideration of the victim's perceptions of the assault cycle and risk factors. However, these factors should be considered cautiously because victim perceptions may be biased. For example, one of the most important determiners of continued contact between a perpetrator and victim is if the perpetrator seeks out treatment. Women are more likely to stay with a batterer that seeks out treatment than one who does not. Given the significant drop out rates and moderate treatment effects for domestic violence programs, a significant increase in the woman's sense of safety simply because the batterer is seeking treatment could be problematic. Nonetheless, research is increasingly suggesting that victim perceptions are integral to risk assessments for domestic violence (Heckert & Gondolf, 2004).

Risk Factors for Domestic Violence

Much of the research has focused on identifying risk factors related to the onset of domestic violence. Furthermore, these risk factors have largely examined physical violence at the exclusion of psychological violence or sexual violence. Though there are some differences between studies depending on the sample and the availability of different factors, these factors can be grouped into demographic and historical factors, psychological factors and relationship factors.

Demographic and historical factors
Demographic and historical factors have long been recognized for their relationship to the onset of domestic violence. Reviews of the literature suggest that age of the perpetrator, socioeconomic status of the perpetrator, race, and childhood exposure to domestic violence form complex relationships with the onset of domestic violence (Feldbau et al., 2000; Holtzworth-Munroe, Smutzler, & Bates, 1997b). Although earlier reviews suggested there was no relationship between age and domestic violence perpetration (Hotaling & Sugarman, 1986), more recent reviews indicate otherwise (Feldbau et al., 2000; Holtzworth-Munroe et al., 1997b). These results have been demonstrated continuously in large national studies and are generally in keeping with the literature on the perpetration of generalized violence. Findings consistently suggest that age is inversely related to the perpetration of domestic violence so that the younger the perpetrator, the greater the risk for domestic violence. In a study focusing on almost 12,000 men enlisted in the military, the authors found that for every 10 years age increased, the risk decreased by 19% that a man would

perpetrate mild violence and 29% for severe violence (Kantor, Jasinski, & Alda-rondo, 1994). These age-related results even hold true when other demographic variables are considered (Kantor et al., 1994).

Socioeconomic status (SES) demonstrates a similar negative or inverse rela-tionship with the perpetration of physical violence in domestic violence conflicts. Furthermore, the most severe levels of aggression appear to be related to lower socioeconomic status (Hotaling & Sugarman, 1990). Socioeconomic status is usually a global variable comprised of multiple variables such as employment status, annual income, education level, and living above or below poverty that indicate overall wealth. Although domestic violence occurs at any economic level, the lower the SES, the greater the risk for the perpetration of domestic violence (Holtzworth-Munroe et al., 1997b). This relationship is continually found for a number of reasons. Individuals from low SES backgrounds are more likely to suffer from a variety of financial and other interpersonal stressors that increase their risk for domestic violence. Individuals from lower SES backgrounds are likely to be less educated. Less educated individuals are less likely to seek out professional assistance and less likely to know where to turn for professional assis-tance when they are in troubled relationships. Because SES is a global variable comprised of many different variables, studies may or may not find a relationship between some of the isolated variables that compose SES. Nevertheless, the rela-tionship between global SES and domestic violence is fairly consistent.

Race and ethnicity also have been related to domestic violence perpetration. Similar to the relationship between SES and domestic violence, there may be some specific racial and ethnic relationships the increase the risk for domestic violence, even though domestic violence cuts across all racial and ethnic groups. Most of the research, as well as many of the largest studies, have found significant differences in the perpetration of domestic violence comparing Caucasians with African-Americans and Hispanics or Latino Americans. Nonetheless, there are a variety of additional factors that can account for these findings. Research has found higher rates of domestic violence in African-Americans (Cazanave & Straus, 1990), Hispanics (Straus & Smith, 1990), and non-Whites in general (Leonard & Blane, 1992). In two large national studies, researchers found that prevalence rates for African-Americans and Latinos were approximately 17% compared to 12% for Caucasians in the same studies (Straus & Gelles, 1986; Straus, Gelles, & Steinmetz, 1980). Studies have even found that African-Ameri-cans are at higher risk for reoffending after initial instances of domestic violence (Mears, Carlson, Holden, & Harris, 2001). However, research has clearly shown that there are a host of other variables that account for these racial and ethnic differences such as economics, education, and social networks (Holtzworth-Munroe et al., 1997b). For example, Benson, Wooldredge, Thistlethwaite, and Fox (2004) found that domestic violence rates vary for African-Americans and Caucasians systematically depending on their community of origin and that racial differences largely disappear when different racial groups reside in similar com-munities. Even though research may suggest a relationship, it is important to realize that other factors account for these apparent racial differences.

A final historical variable that is related to domestic violence perpetration is exposure to domestic violence in one's family of origin. Generally, men who grow up in abusive and violent homes as children are more likely to perpetrate domestic violence. The notion of **intergenerational transmission of violence** has long been a staple of the domestic violence field (Rosenbaum & Leisring, 2003). Intergenerational transmission of violence means that individuals who were exposed to violence as children are more likely to perpetrate violence in their own families as adults. These results are true whether one was physically or verbally abused themselves or witnessed the abuse between others (Barnett & Fagan, 1993; O'Leary & Curley, 1985; Widom, 1989). Mitchell and Finkelhor (2001) even found a 158% increase in the risk for violence if exposed to parental violence as a child. This cycle of violence is self-perpetuating in that individuals who have been abused also are more likely to abuse their own children who are then more likely to abuse their children.

Psychological characteristics related to domestic violence perpetration

There are a host of psychological characteristics that have demonstrated some association with the perpetration of domestic violence such as jealousy, need for power and control, and reduced assertiveness (see Feldbau et al., 2000 for a review). However, research has suggested that there are some psychological characteristics that are more strongly related to the perpetration of domestic violence than others.

One of the most prominent and intuitively appealing psychological characteristics related to domestic violence is the expression of anger or hostility. Although feminist theories for the perpetration of domestic violence are wary of focusing on anger, anger and hostility are often at the core of treatment strategies designed for domestic violence perpetrators. Dutton, Starzomski, and Ryan (1996) compared domestic violence perpetrators and a control group of men on a variety of measures and found that domestic violence perpetrators reported more anger. Hanson, Cadsky, Harris, and Lalonde (1997) further found that anger and hostility scores on a self-report measure differed significantly between severely abusive men, moderately abusive men, and non abusive men. These trends also have been identified across studies using both clinical samples and community samples and were identified as moderate to strong factors for the expression of physical violence (Schumacher, Feldbau et al., 2001; Stith, Smith, Penn, Ward, & Tritt, 2004).

In contrast to the long standing interest in anger and hostility, there is growing interest in the role of substance use and substance abuse in the perpetration of domestic violence (Thompson & Kingree, 2006). Drugs and alcohol have been associated with domestic violence both in terms of chronic abuse and use immediately prior to or during a domestically violent episode. Studies using self-report questionnaires have clearly found that alcohol and drug related problems increase the risk for domestic violence (Cunradi, Caetano, Clark, & Schafer, 1999; Hanson et al., 1997). Moreover, risk also increases with immediate use not simply chronic use. On days in which the perpetrator consumes alcohol, the risk is eight times higher that he will physically assault his partner (Fals-Stewart, 2003) and alcohol consumption is more common in severe violence (38%) than moderate violence (11%) or verbal violence (3%) (Leonard & Quigley, 1999). Accordingly, treatment programs are increasingly examining the impact that substance abuse treatment can have on the perpetration of domestic violence (O'Farrell, Fals-Stewart, Murphy, & Murphy, 2003).

A final psychological characteristic often associated with domestic violence perpetration is depression. At first glance, depression may be counterintuitive to violent behavior but the field is relatively unanimous in finding that perpetrators are more likely to have elevated levels of depression (Stith et al., 2004). Men presenting themselves for marital therapy with their partner differed in their levels of depressive symptoms with martially violent men reporting more depression than non violent men (Boyle & Vivian, 1996). In one study, nearly two-thirds of the domestic violence perpetrators were depressed compared to only one-third of the rest of the sample (Maiuro, Cahn, Vitaliano, Wagner, & Zegree, 1988). Depression may be related to a heightened display of emotion that is characteristic of at least some batterers (Holtzworth-Munroe and Stuart, 1994). These batterers are likely to exhibit borderline tendencies, exhibit heightened levels of depression and express more suicidal ideas and behavior (Dutton, 2002).

Relationship and contextual factors related to perpetration

Another extremely important area to consider for potential risk factors is the relationship itself. Individuals who are unhappy or dissatisfied with their relationship, frequently argue with their partner, and demonstrate psychological aggression are at increased risk for the perpetration of domestic violence (Feldbau-Kohn et al., 2000). There are even specific communication patterns that suggest increase risk (Holtzworth-Munroe et al., 1997b). In fact, relationship factors may be among the best predictors of domestic violence (Stith et al., 2004).

It is not surprisingly that couples report less satisfaction with abusive relationships than nonabusive relationships but it is important that marital satisfaction of the perpetrator is itself predictive of violence toward his partner. There appears to be a clear association between violence and relationship dissatisfaction. Julian and McKenry (1993) found a significant predictive relationship between reported satisfaction with their relationship and self-reported violence in a group of men presenting for treatment. However, the evidence for a predictive relationship between marital satisfaction and violence is not as clear. The question becomes one of the chicken versus the egg. Does the violence decrease marital satisfaction or does decreased marital satisfaction lead to violence? Results from one of the few longitudinal studies addressing the issue suggest a more complex relationship. O'Leary, Malone, and Tyree (1994) found that marital dissatisfaction after 18 months of marriage did not predict later physical aggression. However, marital dissatisfaction at 18 months predicted psychological aggression, which predicted physical aggression at 30 months after marriage.

Self-reported marital satisfaction may be as important as the communication patterns couples exhibit with one another. This research has focused both on observational studies of couples and interviews. In many studies, couples are videotaped discussing their relationship or problems in their relationship. Researchers later observe these interactions in detail and identify several aspects of these conversations that increase the risk for future physical violence. Husbands who exhibit physical aggression are more likely to dismiss their partners' opinion, threaten or mimic their gestures, become defensive and use negative physical contact than verbally aggressive husbands (Margolin, Bruman, & John, 1989; Margolin, John, & Gleberman, 1989). Studies examining self-report data also have found that violent couples are more likely to use more verbal attacks, more anger, and are more likely to withdraw from the situation (Lloyd, 1990).

Other characteristics related to domestic violence perpetration
In addition to these routine aspects of intimate relationships, there also appear to be some risk factors that are less intuitive. Specifically, there are two events that significantly increase the risk for relationship violence. First, evidence suggests that pregnancy significantly increases risk for domestic violence and that a significant number of women begin to be victimized during pregnancy (Jasinski & Kantor, 2001). Another period of time during the relationship that is especially dangerous for women is at the ending of the relationship. One study showed the end of an intimate relationship to be the most dangerous time for women because their partners become threatened by a clear indication of a change or loss in the relationship (Wilson, Johnson, & Daly, 1995).

So far we have focused on physical aggression in identifying factors related to domestic violence. However, as already discussed, there are a variety of forms of domestic violence including psychological aggression, sexual aggression and even the most severe consequence, homicide. Very few studies have identified the risk factors for sexual abuse in domestic violence situations. Black, Heyman, and Slep (2001) reviewed the available studies and found several risk factors for sexual abuse. Victims under 30 and over 50 are at greater risk, who come from low SES backgrounds, who were sexually assaulted outside of the relationship, and who have experienced severe physical aggression in general (Black et al., 2001). Although more difficult to predict than physical violence, Schumacher, Slep, and Heyman (2001) concluded that relationship variables such as the communication patterns previously described along with perpetrator characteristics (i.e., anger, borderline personality characteristics, passive–aggressive characteristics, and self-defeating characteristics) indicated higher risk for psychological abuse. Surprisingly, SES and witnessing violence as a child are unrelated to psychological abuse in a relationship.

An area of increasing concern is the occurrence of homicide in domestically violence relationships. For example, **femicide** is the leading cause of premature death for women in the United States (Greenfield et al., 1998). Research suggests that there are unique as well as consistent risk factors for cases of homicide. A history of domestic violence and a presence of handguns appear to be the strongest risk factors for intimate partner homicide with the ending of a relationship also serving as a strong predictor (Campbell, Sharps, & Glass, 2001). In addition, generalized violence, alcohol abuse, unemployment, and being a member of a racial minority are significant risk factors for homicide (Campbell et al., 2001). One of the most comprehensive studies of intimate partner homicide was conducted across 11 cities and included information from 220 female victims. Results showed that relationships in which the perpetrator had access to a gun, the perpetrator made prior threats with a weapon, the perpetrator's stepchild was in the home, and the parties were separated were at greater risk. Never living together and prior domestic violence arrests were protective factors for homicide (Campbell et al., 2003).

Assessing Risk and Recidivism

In addition to those factors related to the onset of domestic violence, research has also focused on factors related to recidivism. Hilton and Harris (2005) argue that the most relevant risk factors are general antisocial behavior, psychopathy, substance abuse, a history of assault, and psychological abuse in the relationship. Cattaneo and Goodman (2005) agreed with some of Hilton and Harris' review but also focused on additional interpersonal (e.g., length of time lived together) and systemic factors (e.g., stake in conforming their behavior to societal expectations) that are relevant to domestic violence recidivism. Examinations of risk factors specifically for recidivism is relatively recent and a great deal of research is needed to assess these factors in comparison to factors related to the onset of abuse. However, several measures have been devised based on the general risk factor literature and the literature focusing on recidivism. Nonetheless, information regarding the effectiveness of these measures is only beginning to accrue.

Available risk assessment measures for domestic violence
As mentioned previously, there are several aspects of risk assessment within domestic violence that are similar to general risk assessment but there are also differences because of the nature of domestic violence. Whittemore and Kropp (2002) identified five principles of risk assessment that forensic psychologists should be aware of in a domestic violence context. First, they recommend that risk assessment should consider risk factors supported in the literature. This recommendation is in keeping with general risk assessment and possible because of the growing literature on risk factors for domestic violence. Second, they recommend that domestic violence risk assessments should use multiple sources of information. Not only is this recommendation in keeping with the overall risk assessment literature but it also is consistent with the focus of assessment described in Chapter 2 and the importance of converging evidence. Therefore, an interview with the defendant, a review of police records, and interview with the victim are strongly encouraged. Whittemore and Kropp (2002) pay special mention in the third principle of making sure risk assessments are victim-informed. This step is especially important if the perpetrator and victim plan on continuing their relationship or must associate with one another because they share children. Given that perpetrators also may be less than truthful,

final type of stalker is the erotomanic stalker who is characterized by delusional beliefs in an already existing relationship with an idealized victim. Erotomanic stalkers include about 5% of all stalkers. Meloy's subtypes are theoretical but empirical research supported some of these distinctions.

After more attention began to be placed on stalking and it became clear that the majority of stalkers had a significant intimate relationship with their victims (Sfiligoj, 2003), the natural association between stalking and domestic violence was explored. Douglas and Dutton (2001) argue that most stalkers are similar to the borderline/dysphoric batterers identified by Holtzworth-Munroe and Stuart (1994). They share the extreme emotional dysregulation in terms of depression, anger, jealousy, and substance abuse and are further likely to have

Box 10.2.   Celebrity Stalkers from *My Sister Sam* to David Letterman

When most people think of stalkers they tend to think of the high profile celebrity stalkers and the extreme measures they take to express their obsessive tendencies toward their victims. For example, Madonna was stalked by a man who scaled the wall of her home, threatened to cut her throat, and came within feet of her. David Letterman was stalked by a woman who continually broke into his Connecticut home, stole his car and claimed to be his wife when stopped by a law enforcement officer, and was arrested for shoplifting near his mother's house in Indiana. However, one of the original celebrity stalking cases that ended tragically but contributed immensely to the public and legal awareness about stalking occurred in 1989.

Rebecca Schaeffer was the star of a short lived sit-com in the 1980s called *My Sister Sam* and was seen as an up and coming young star in Hollywood before she was murdered. Schaeffer's killer, Robert Bardo, began stalking her by writing her letters as any other fan would. He even showed up at the gates of the studio where *My Sister Sam* was being taped with roses and a Teddy bear but he was turned away. The stalking escalated though when he showed up at the studio again with a concealed knife but was

once again denied entry. He then started to write Schaeffer love letter after love letter, collected videos of all of her television appearances, plastered his room with her picture, and made comments to his friends and family that if he could not have her then nobody would. He became relentless in his mission to meet her doing such things as calling her agent for her address, walking the streets of Los Angeles asking random passersby if they knew where the woman in the picture he showed them lived, and finally he successfully hired a private detective to get her address. Bardo showed up at Schaeffer's apartment and rang the bell of her apartment building entrance one fateful day. The intercom in her apartment was not working so she came down to the entrance where Bardo handed her a picture expressing his admiration of her. Schaeffer asked him to leave but he later rang the buzzer again and hid so she could not see that it was him until she opened the door. When she did open the door, Bardo shot her in the chest twice and walked away. Schaeffer's tragic death is frequently identified as one of the impetuses for legislation designed to prevent stalking and for formation of a special Los Angeles Police Department unit focused largely on stalking.

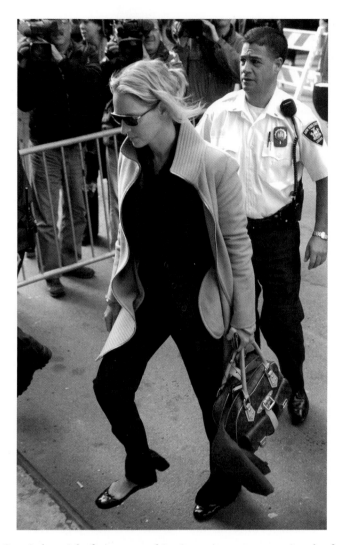

Figure 10.2. A lovesick former psychiatric patient was convicted of stalking and harassing actress Uma Thurman in May 2008. Dennis Van Tine.

suffered childhood trauma and poor emotional attachment to their care givers. Research also reveals that the severity of domestic violence experienced in an intimate relationship is related to future stalking (Logan, Leukefeld, & Walker, 2000).

Stalking generally is comprised of a variety of different behaviors that can include minor behaviors such as following the victim, leaving unwanted phone calls, sending unwanted gifts to more serious behaviors of making threats or damaging property (Langhinrichsen-Rohling, Palarea, Cohen, & Rohling, 2000). However, the most prevalent stalking activities appear to consist of following, spying, or standing outside the victims home (77%), unwanted phone calls (52%), overt threats (52%), sent unwanted letters or items (30%), vandalization of property (29.5%), and killing or threatening pets (7.5%). Unlike some of the research on domestic violence perpetration in general, the overwhelming majority of victims tend to be women (78%) and the overwhelming number of perpetrators are men (87%). In addition, women are more likely to have a prior relationship with their stalker and overall about 25% to 40% of stalkers physically assault their victims. Some of the risk markers for stalking include extreme jealousy and possessiveness, need for control, and absence of friends of their own, and poor social skills (Tjaden & Thoeness, 1998).

Summary

Domestic violence can take on many forms including physical aggression, sexual aggression, and even psychological aggression. The Conflict Tactics Scale (CTS) is the most common measure used to assess domestic violence in all its forms, though most of the research and clinical practice focus on physical aggression. The precise form of aggression and even the method used to assess it are important in evaluating the wide range of prevalence figures for domestic violence. Studies focusing on community samples in which subjects may be randomly telephoned are going to reveal much lower prevalence rates than studies focusing on couples seeking therapy for marital problems. No matter the source of the research or the methods employed, it is very clear that domestic violence is a significant problem.

Although the CTS is the most commonly employed measure to assess the frequency and severity of domestic violence, there have been criticisms of the measure and the manner in which it is used. For example, research has revealed that women report lower rates of domestic violence than their male partners using the CTS and many argue that the CTS fails to take into account the context in which the domestic violence occurs. The CTS does not assess the consequences of domestic violence well, which are significant and varied. In addition to the physical injuries that result from physical aggression, victims often suffer from posttraumatic stress disorder, depression, and lowered self-esteem. Moreover, it may well be the psychological abuse that is more likely to lead to these psychological consequences than physical abuse.

A number of risk factors have been identified for the perpetration of physical aggression. These risk factors include demographic and historical factors, psychological characteristics, and relationship and contextual factors. Demographic factors commonly related to domestic violence include age, socioeconomic status, race and ethnicity, and exposure to violence as a child. The major psychological characteristics related to the perpetration of domestic violence are anger and hostility, substance abuse, and depression. Reduced marital satisfaction, specific communication patterns, and specific relationship events are also related to the perpetration of domestic violence.

There are some unique aspects to risk assessment involving domestic violence and even specific risk factors for recidivism that differ from the risk factors related to the onset of physical, sexual, or psychological aggression. There also are several risk assessment instruments designed specifically for the assessment of domestic violence risk. The SARA, DAS, and ODARA are three measures and each offers a unique perspective to the assessment of risk. However, none of them has extensive research supporting its use and caution should be exercised in using them.

There are a variety of different interventions that have been designed to reduce or eliminate domestic violence. These interventions include psychological and educational programs for perpetrators, victims, and even couples along with community and criminal justice interventions. No single approach can reduce domestic violence in itself. The best approach to reducing domestic violence is a comprehensive or multimodal approach that encourages use of psychological, community, and legal approaches to the problem.

Because much of the focus in domestic violence research and practice has been on male perpetration, female perpetration of domestic violence has long been controversial. Much of the controversy is probably the result of the contrast in the professional experiences of individuals working with battered women in shelters and the feminist explanations for domestic violence with the literature suggesting equal rates of perpetration. Research suggests that these contrasting views are likely the result of the samples used and that while men and women probably exhibit equal frequency rates, the injuries resulting from the aggression are not equal.

A final area associated with domestic violence is stalking of intimate partners. Although stalking is often associated with high profile celebrity cases, the majority of stalking takes place within a past or present intimate relationship. Furthermore, it may be that these stalking instances are also the most dangerous for the person being stalked. Stalking can consist of a variety of unwanted behaviors such as leaving letters, following, repeated phone calls, direct threats, or even property damage. Research has also began to identify some preliminary risk markers for stalking.

Key Terms

battering	intergenerational transmission of violence
clinical sample	mandatory arrests
community sample	restraining order
femicide	

Further Readings

Dutton, D. G. (2007). *The abusive personality: Violence and control in intimate relationships* (2nd ed.). New York: Guilford Press.

Gelles, R. J. (1997). *Intimate violence in families* (3rd ed.). Thousand Oaks, CA: Sage Publications, Inc.

11

Juvenile Delinquency and Juvenile Justice

Greater media attention to crimes involving children, especially school shootings and other violent crimes has increased the attention placed upon the juvenile justice system and juvenile delinquency (Krisberg & Wolf, 2005). Historically, childhood has been a distinctive period in the development of human beings where future adults were shaped and lessons learned that would impact the rest of their lives. The view of a distinctive period between childhood and adulthood, adolescence, is a more recent development. Adolescents are considered more advanced than children and able to accept some of the responsibility that occurs in adulthood like driving a car or holding a job. Regardless, they are not adults and not afforded all the rights of adults. Adolescents are typically the focus of juvenile interventions. This focus occurs not only because they often commit delinquent behaviors and serious violent behaviors but also because most jurisdictions specifically bar children, completely before age seven, from culpability for any delinquent or criminal behavior. Although the word juvenile refers to any child under the age of majority, most of the research and resources of the juvenile system focus on adolescents.

Special detention centers were established in many places in Europe before the nineteenth century, and juvenile courts were first established at the turn of the twentieth century in the United States, built squarely on the notion that children were different than adults. Policy makers believed that if adolescents committed societal transgressions, they should not be punished as adults but instead rehabilitated because there was still time to prevent them from leading antisocial lives as adults. However, society has become increasingly concerned about the perceived increase in the frequency and severity of crime committed by children and adolescents. Some of this perception has been fueled by sensationalized crimes committed by juveniles such as the death of a young girl while her playmate was reportedly practicing professional wrestling moves (Box. 11.1). Even prior to the advent of this view, the courts were beginning to think that juvenile courts should be more similar to adult criminal courts and protect

Box 11.1.   Juvenile Violence: The Youngest Person Ever Sentenced to Life in Prison

Many of the public perceptions that juvenile violence has been increasing dramatically are fueled by public awareness of high profile crimes such as the death of Tiffany Eunick in 1999. Kathleen Grossett-Tate was watching six year-old Tiffany one evening, the child of a friend, along with her 12-year-old son, Lionel Tate. Toward the end of the evening Ms. Tate went upstairs to rest. Lionel later came to wake her up reporting that Tiffany had stopped breathing. After Tiffany's death, Lionel was charged with her murder.

The case made national headlines in the United States after Lionel and his attorneys claimed that Tiffany had died as a result of the 170 lb Lionel practicing professional wrestling moves on the 45 lb Tiffany. Prosecution experts testified that her injuries were brutal and could not have occurred as Lionel claimed. After Lionel's mother turned down a plea bargain that would have resulted in him serving a three year sentence, Lionel was convicted and became the youngest person in the United States to be sentenced to death. Tate's conviction was overturned in 2004 because he was not evaluated for competency to stand trial. This result allowed his attorneys to accept the original plea bargain and Lionel Tate served his sentence under house arrest and received 10 years probation. However, this incident was not the end of his criminal involvement. Tate violated his probation the same year he accepted the plea bargain because he left his house carrying a knife. He received an additional 5 years of probation but was once again arrested and charged with holding up a pizza delivery man with a gun. Lionel Tate was sentenced to 30 years in prison in May 2006 for the incident. Horrific cases such as Tate's often lead the public to believe juvenile violence is out of control.

juveniles by affording them the same rights that adults received in the adversarial criminal courts. Changing views of the courts and the general public led to some gray areas in dealing with juveniles. Could they be rehabilitated and should that be the goal of the juvenile courts, given some of the serious crimes being committed by juveniles? At what age are juveniles as responsible for their crimes as adults? How could any of these answers be determined?

As a result, the juvenile justice system has received a great deal of attention and undergone some significant changes in the latter part of the twentieth century and the early part of the twenty-first century. The role of the forensic psychologist has changed greatly in a context in which some questioned whether the role of mental health professionals was already too expansive (Melton et al., 1997). Some of the duties we have talked about in terms of adults such as competency and insanity were unheard of in the juvenile court but now have become more common. In addition, changes in the law intended to give juveniles the **due process** protections common in adult criminal matters also may have discouraged the rehabilitation model juvenile courts were founded upon. This change occurred while public perception, which has not always matched the reality, has been that juvenile crime and specifically juvenile violence is increasing and that there is a greater need to punish juveniles instead of rehabilitating them. This chapter will examine delinquent or antisocial behavior committed by juveniles in the context of the evolving juvenile court and the overall changes that have made it more likely for juveniles to be tried as adults. We will also pay specific attention to contemporary issues such as school violence and school shootings.

History of the Juvenile Court

The first juvenile court was established in 1899 and juvenile courts have spread to almost every industrialized country in the world (Zimring, 2000a). Immediately, the juvenile courts were distinguished from their adult counterparts. The focus of the juvenile justice system was on the rehabilitation of juveniles, not on their conviction and punishment. Juveniles were viewed as not fully responsible for their acts and in need of assistance to avoid a continued life of adult criminal behavior. The focus on rehabilitation instead of punishment meant that the court did not concentrate on the offense but on the offender. Practically, this meant a juvenile was not automatically punished more harshly for a severe transgression than for a minor one. If a juvenile committed a minor crime but was in need of a number of different services that the juvenile court could offer such as academic assistance, adult supervision, or mental health treatment, she would receive it. A juvenile who stole the hubcaps off a neighbor's car was more likely to compensate the neighbor for the hubcaps by working for the money than be incarcerated because he had broken the law. It was believed that such a practice would teach the juvenile a lesson and that incarceration was not the most effective or cost-efficient way to prevent recidivism.

Juvenile proceedings were not adversarial because the child was not only being punished but being cared for by a judge who had broad discretion in rendering decisions (Steffen & Ackerman, 1999). This approach was based on the legal notion of parens patriae (Chapter 9). The juvenile courts believed they had a responsibility to protect and take care of juvenile offenders and therefore took additional steps like closing the proceedings to outsiders and sealing juvenile records. Many of the offenses that brought juveniles before the juvenile courts were status offenses. Status offenses are offenses that could only be committed by juveniles such as truancy and running away from home. They are not viewed as crimes but as juvenile offenses. Generally, juveniles were perceived as lacking culpability for their offenses. Any child under age seven clearly was not responsible and it was believed that children from 7 to 14 were not able to form criminal intent (Otto & Borum, 2003).

From the early intent of the juvenile system, it is easy to see the implications for therapeutic jurisprudence. In fact, it could be argued that the early juvenile system embodied the precise notion of therapeutic jurisprudence. The juvenile courts were established to be different from the traditional punitive approach taken in the adult criminal courts; they were established to be therapeutic. The juvenile court intended to be rehabilitative by focusing on the needs of the children and the personal and environmental factors leading to their delinquent behavior. By doing so, they believed that children would be less likely to commit additional crimes, less likely to exhibit problematic behavior and more likely to become productive members of society. However, many questioned whether the courts fell short of their intended rehabilitative goals and whether it was appropriate to treat juveniles different, especially at the cost of many of the constitutional rights adults were afforded.

The juvenile courts in the United States began to change in the 1960s. In *Kent v. United States* (1966) the Supreme Court argued that juveniles received the worst of the juvenile system and the adult system. They were not given either the due process safeguards of adults or the benefits of treatment that children were suppose to receive. *Kent* formally recognized the right of juveniles to have the assistance of counsel if they faced criminal charges. Another case, *In re Gault* (1967) indicated the Court's skepticism of the juvenile system more explicitly (Box 11.2). The Supreme Court clearly stated that juveniles were persons to be protected under the Bill of Rights and that they should be

Box 11.2.   Altering the Juvenile Justice System: *In re Gault*

In re Gault (1967) has been considered one of the most important, if not the most important, cases in the history of juvenile law. Despite its unique impact on the juvenile justice system, *In re Gault* involved a fairly common set of circumstances. Gerald Gault was a 15 year-old boy who was on probation for accompanying another boy who had stolen a wallet. In June 1964, he was taken into custody by local law enforcement officers with his friend, Ronald Lewis. A neighbor had complained to police that Gault and his friend were making obscene and lewd phone calls to her residence. When Gault was arrested his parents were not home and the officers did not leave any notice at the home that Gault had been taken into custody. Gault's parents only learned of his arrest after his mother arrived home early that evening and sent their older son to check on Gault's whereabouts.

After eventually contacting the appropriate authority, his mother was told a hearing would take place on the following day. At the hearing there were no witnesses sworn in, including the complaining witness, and Gault was not given an attorney nor were any of his rights explained. Eventually, Gault was committed to a state school until he was 21 years-old. On appeal, it was argued that the procedures used to commit him to the facility were unconstitutional and violated several of his due process rights. The United States Supreme Court agreed and held that juveniles should be given due process rights as adults, receive written notice of any court proceedings, be advised of their right to counsel, be advised of their right against self-incrimination, and given the right of sworn testimony of their accusers and to cross examine them.

Table 11.1.   Differences in the United States Juvenile and Adult Systems

	Juvenile system	Adult system
Detention	Taken into custody	Arrested
Culpability	Found or adjudicated delinquent	Found guilty
Disposition	Committed or placed	Incarcerated
Presence of jury	No right to a jury trial	Right to a jury trial
Treatment	Right to treatment	No right to treatment
Proceedings	Informal	Formal
Status offenses	Recognized	Not recognized
Death penalty	Does not apply	Applicable in capital offenses
Official record	Sealed	Permanent

Source: Adapted from Shoemaker and Wolfe (2005)

given due process (*In re Gault*, 1967). Though these cases required that juveniles receive some of the due process rights long considered essential to adult criminal defendants, they also began to suggest that the divide between adults and children was not as wide as had been previously thought.

Beginning in the 1980s and 1990s, almost every state in the United States changed their juvenile statutes to reduce the emphasis on rehabilitation (Zimring, 1998) and create more of a balance between rehabilitation and punishment. These changes were due in part to the public perception that juvenile crime was dramatically increasing. The de-emphasis of rehabilitation was marked by several procedural trends. The upper age range was frequently lowered for jurisdiction over a juvenile. For example, previously a juvenile court may have responsibility for supervision of a child until he or she turned 21 years of age but many states reduced that age from 21 to 16. Certain serious offenses automatically became the responsibility of the criminal courts. Age ranges for transfer to criminal court were expanded downward so that when previously only children as young as 16 could be subject to criminal courts, children as young as 14 or 12 may be transferred from juvenile court to adult criminal court. Juvenile commitments also were extended into adult criminal sentences instead of expiring when the juvenile reached a particular maximum age. However, there still remain important differences in terminology and practice between the juvenile and adult systems of justice (Table 11.1) (Shoemaker & Wolfe, 2005).

Processing in the Juvenile Courts

Although there are variations across different jurisdictions, the processing of juveniles through the juvenile court systems shares a number of similarities across the United Kingdom, Canada, and the United States (Hoge & Andrews,

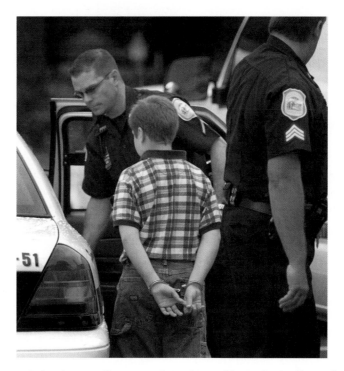

Figure 11.1.   Gabriel Keys (foreground) is arrested by police officers for trespassing in Pinellas Park, Florida, March 23, 2005. © REUTERS/Carlos Barria

1996). The process normally begins with some sort of law enforcement contact. The contact may be the result of a complaint by a parent, a school, or a member of the public and can lead to a variety of legal outcomes, even at this stage. Law enforcement can choose to question, release, release with a warning, take children into custody, or detain them for an extended period of time (see Figure 11.1). Normally, it is frowned upon to hold a child with adult offenders but in some jurisdictions there may not be separate juvenile facilities and in these instances there are often legal requirements that prohibit extensive incarceration near adult offenders. If a juvenile is formally charged or brought into custody, some sort of intake normally follows. Juvenile intakes are usually performed by officers from the juvenile probation office or prosecutors. They consist of an examination of the specifics of the alleged offense and whether there is sufficient evidence to move forward with the allegation or dismiss the case. There is considerable variation across different jurisdictions regarding the specifics of this process. If the determination is made to go forward after the initial intake, the adjudication process continues. Juveniles may be detained prior to their case being formally adjudicated but juveniles can be held over for a juvenile hearing to determine their guilt or innocence, transferred to criminal court, or again the charges could be dismissed at this stage. If the juvenile continued in the juvenile court, a hearing is normally scheduled to determine the outcome or disposition of the case (Hoge & Andrews, 1996).

Prior to the disposition of the case, the probation officer normally prepares a formal report to assist the court. If the court determines the juvenile is delinquent, this report serves as the basis for formulating any intervention plan for the juvenile. For example, the probation officer may have detected through his investigation that the juvenile is often unsupervised and routinely truant from school. Part of the plan could be to mandate that the child attend school regularly or face additional penalties and require the juvenile to participate in an after school activity. If the juvenile is found to be delinquent, the judge identifies sanctions and may order additional evaluations to better inform the court about a possible disposition of the case. For example, the initial report from the probation officer may have suggested some possible mental health needs. The judge may require the juvenile undergo a psychological evaluation to further examine the necessity of psychotherapy or psychiatric treatment. Once the judge has determined the final sanctions necessary, the juvenile must follow the judge's orders. These orders may consist of restitution to the victim, obtaining a job, attending therapy, reporting to the probation officer, abstention from drugs and alcohol with regular drug testing or even incarceration in a juvenile detention center. The length and conditions of the probation may be determined at this time or more likely open ended and dependent on the juvenile meeting all of the conditions of their probation (Roberts, 2004). Typically, once juveniles have met all the conditions of their probation they are released from the authority of the juvenile court unless there are additional concerns or new charges filed. This description only provides a broad outline and specific jurisdictions may slightly alter this process or even depart significantly from it. However, in most instances these steps are characteristic of the process involved in moving a juvenile through the juvenile court system.

Juvenile Delinquency and Juvenile Offenses

What exactly is meant by the term **juvenile delinquency**? Juvenile delinquency is frequently used to describe behavior that is a violation of criminal law but is committed by individuals who have not yet become adults. The nature of juvenile offenses is varied and can include anything from status offenses to murder. Moreover, the public's view of these crimes often contrasts with the realities. The Department of Justice is a common source for crime statistics in the United States and has reported that juvenile crime is at its lowest in 20 years (U.S. Department of Justice, 2001). There has been a 30% decrease in sexual assaults, 68% decrease in murders, a 53% drop in robberies, a 39% drop in weapons related arrests, and a 24% drop in aggravated assaults committed by juveniles (Snyder, 2000). Even at its highest point, less than 6% of youths under eighteen years of age have ever been arrested and less than 10% of juveniles who have committed crimes have committed violent crimes (Snyder, 2000). Nonetheless, the public generally believes there has been a significant increase in juvenile crime. This belief may be partially a result of the increase in news coverage on juvenile crime, despite the decreased prevalence (Dorfman & Schiraldi, 2001). It seems like stories about the next Columbine are a frequent part of the news.

Despite the good news that there seems to be an overall trend for a decrease in the juvenile crime rate, there are some problems and distressing trends. Overall, there are about 2 million juvenile arrests each year, 1 million are sent to juvenile court, about 500,000 are admitted to detention centers, and about 10,000 of these juveniles are sent to criminal court for further adjudication (Shoemaker & Wolfe, 2005). About 61% of juvenile proceedings are delinquency proceedings, 19% for status offenses, and 19% for victimization or abuse of children (Ostrom, Kauder, & LaFountain, 2001). Research is indicating a distressing number of juvenile offenders are younger and that more juvenile cases are being sent to adult courts (Sickmund, 1994). Specifically, 58% of all juveniles are younger than 16 years of age, 32% are younger than 15 years old, and 9% are 12 and younger (Snyder & Sickmund, 1999; U. S. Department of Justice, 2001). These figures are especially problematic because the younger a juvenile offender is, the more likely he is to commit more violent and more serious offenses than juveniles who initially offend at a later age (Cottle, Lee, & Heilbrun, 2001). Furthermore, a dramatic increase in juvenile crime has occurred among girls. Overall, there has been an 83% increase in female juvenile crime (Snyder, 2000). The rise in juvenile crimes among females is at least partially the result of the runaways who turn to shoplifting, prostitution, and drug offenses to cope with living on the streets (Henriques & Manatu-Rupert, 2001).

One type of juvenile offense not typically seen as a serious offense but often identified as a gateway for serious offenses are status offenses. Curfew and loitering violations more than doubled from 1993 to 1997 but then declined 17% by 1999 (Snyder, 2000). Although these crimes are less serious, there are few opportunities for rehabilitation because of the increased focus on more serious offenders and punitive interventions for less antisocial juveniles. Placement of juvenile status offenders then becomes problematic because the juvenile court does not want to encourage continued antisocial behavior by placing them in situations where they may be exposed to negative peer influences. If the court places a young juvenile, who has committed a relatively minor offense, in a juvenile detention center there is a risk that he will begin to associate with individuals who are more antisocial and adopt their antisocial behavior.

Another significant area of juvenile delinquency is the commission of property crime. Property crimes typically include offenses like burglary, theft, and arson. About one-third of all juvenile arrests are for a property-related crime (Godwin & Helms, 2002). Burglary is often characterized by entering a structure of some kind and unlawfully stealing property on those premises. Burglary accounts for about one-quarter of all juvenile offenses (Snyder & Sickmund, 1999). Theft is defined as the unlawful taking or possession of property and differs from burglary in that the offender has entered a dwelling or is around the property legally, it is the taking of the property that is illegal. Theft would

two processes because it necessitates a clear understanding of the context in which the juvenile will function (Grisso, 2003c).

Competency Evaluations

The competence of a juvenile was rarely an issue in the juvenile courts when rehabilitation was the focus, but as there has been recognition of the courts' more punitive stance, forensic psychologists have increasingly been called upon to perform competency evaluations. As discussed (Chapter 8), criminal competency normally focuses on ensuring that the defendant understands the proceedings and the potential consequences of any legal decisions. Competency is normally raised for juveniles in regard to competency to stand trial (Bonnie & Grisso, 2000) but also can be an issue in regard to understanding their Miranda rights (Grisso, 2003c). Issues related to competency become especially difficult to determine in regard to juveniles because of their immaturity and underdeveloped cognitive abilities and the disposition of a case where incompetence is due to developmental issues. However, most competency statutes do not include developmental or psychosocial immaturity as an important issue. Florida is one state that specifically does incorporate the notion into its competency statutes for juveniles. The idea of developmental immaturity is important because in adult criminal cases, the defendant would be held for restoration of competence but with a juvenile that may mean waiting for them to grow and mature into adulthood. Some research even suggests that many juvenile offenders, especially those under 14, are not competent to stand trial (Steinberg et al., 2003) and that psychosocial immaturity is very important in assessing the competence of a juvenile (Grisso et al., 2003c). As a result of the lack of legal criteria and uncertainty, there continues to be discussion about whether competency should even be raised as an issue for juveniles (Zimring, 2000b).

Ryba, Cooper, and Zapf (2003) surveyed psychologists to gather some idea of the most commonly employed methods used in these situations. In their survey of 82 forensic psychologists who had expertise in juvenile forensic assessment, there were seven areas that at least 70% of the respondents indicated as essential in conducting a juvenile competency to stand trial evaluation. These essential areas included: evaluation of current mental status (95.1%); understanding the charges or penalties (95.1%); competency to stand trial related abilities (91.5%); capacity to participate with attorney (90.2%); mental illness opinion (86.6%); understanding of the trial process (85.4%); and mental illness/mental retardation/immaturity rationale (74.4%). Results were extremely similar to those found in previous research surveying forensic psychologists in regard to adult competency (Borum & Grisso, 1996). Respondents also were asked questions about the use of different psychological tests and specialized forensic tests. There was much less consensus in regard to the specific tests used even though 79% of the respondents believed in psychological testing and 70% thought forensic testing was essential or recommended in juvenile competency evaluations (Ryba et al., 2003). These results suggest there is some consensus in regard to the practice that occurs in juvenile competency evaluations but there is little research to assist forensic psychologists in knowing whether these more common practices are empirically justified.

Insanity Evaluations

Another area where it was almost unheard of for forensic psychologists to practice in juvenile court was in determining criminal responsibility or insanity. It is interesting that historically many jurisdictions have ruled that any child under seven, and even under 11 in some jurisdictions, automatically do not have the required mens rea or guilty mind in order to commit a criminal act for which they can be held responsible (Tanenhaus, 2000). Nevertheless, as juveniles were afforded more due process rights and the punitive nature of the juvenile courts were recognized, forensic psychologists were needed to evaluate whether juveniles were insane at the time of a delinquent act.

As is the case with competency, there is little empirical basis for the evaluation of a juvenile's mental state at the time of the offense (i.e., insanity) and there are not any measures designed especially for juveniles. Therefore, it has been recommended that forensic psychologists rely on those procedures developed for adult criminals (Otto & Borum, 2003). However, the forensic psychologist has the added burden of distinguishing the delinquent behavior not only from a potential mental illness but also the juvenile's own immaturity. Although it is clear that insanity has been raised in regard to juveniles with added frequency, it is still extremely rare (Haller, 2000). Some states have even ruled that juveniles are not entitled to an insanity defense. Furthermore, even if a state allows for the defense many still do not have a formal process set up for handling juveniles acquitted NGRI.

Risk Assessment

A final area, in which forensic psychologists are increasingly being used in juvenile courts, is risk assessment. Risk assessment is of course an issue that is intertwined with other roles such as the evaluation of treatment amenability and transfer to criminal court. However, it also represents a distinct role performed by forensic psychologists in this context and can be an important issue at almost every stage of the juvenile system (Otto & Borum, 2003). Assessment of risk in juveniles is significantly different from risk assessment with adults because of the dynamic nature of youth. Juveniles are continually developing and changing and do not offer the years of stability from which clear static risk factors can be identified.

Another form of risk assessment frequently employed with juveniles is **threat assessment**. Threat assessment occurs when a juvenile comes to the attention of those in authority through certain behaviors or verbalizations that suggest he or she is a threat to commit future violence (Randazzo et al., 2006). One context in which threat assessment occurs that we will discuss in more detail later is school violence or school shootings. In this context, the forensic psychologist must evaluate whether the juvenile poses a serious threat to act out in the future because he is exhibiting certain characteristics that suggest he is following a particular developmental course.

However, the majority of risk assessments are of the traditional variety. There are several structured or actuarial instruments that have been developed for juveniles. Two of the more notable instruments are the Early Assessment Risk List (EARL) for girls and boys (Augimeri, Koegl, Webster, & Levene, 2001) and the Structured Assessment of Violence Risk in Youth (SAVRY; Bartel, Borum, & Forth, 2000). These tools are designed to identify the most relevant risk factors and then encourage the forensic psychologist to rate the juvenile on the presence of the characteristics captured in each risk factor. Although the procedures and use of structured approaches to risk assessment are similar in juveniles and adults, it is important to recognize there are differences. A forensic psychologist performing a juvenile risk assessment needs to be aware of the developmental nature of both delinquent behavior and normal juvenile behavior (Borum, 2003). This task, combined with the lack of wide scale empirical support for any juvenile risk assessment tool, makes it especially difficult for the forensic psychologist to perform risk assessments on juveniles.

Special Issues in Regard to Juveniles: School Violence

As Borum (2000) states, "despite recent declines in the reported rates of juvenile violence, there appears to be increasing public and professional concern about violent behavior among children and adolescents" (p. 1263). Borum's quote sums up much of the current chapter and the state of the research and practice in regard to juveniles. Even though we know juvenile violence has decreased, we continue to be very interested in it, as seen in the increasing media attention and even in the call for forensic psychologists to participate more in the evaluation and treatment of youth, especially violent youth. Part of the increased attention is not just the perception that juveniles are becoming more dangerous but that they are doing so in the location that parents thought they would be the safest, the schools. As a result of the specter of juvenile violence and juvenile murder, there have been increasing calls for more punitive approaches to handling violent juveniles.

School Violence and School Shootings

Increasing public concern about school violence largely has been fueled by and become associated with student-perpetrated shootings in such places as Paducah, Kentucky; Jonesboro, Arkansas, and Columbine High School in Colorado during the 1990s. Fears that arose after these early shootings have only been reinforced by more recent shootings at Dawson College in Montreal, Canada where one student was killed and more than a dozen were wounded and the

Box 11.3. The Virginia Tech Tragedy: Its Role in School Shootings and Forensic Psychology

On April 16, 2007 the single largest school shooting in the history of the United States took place at Virginia Tech University. Thirty-two people were killed and 25 were wounded in two separate attacks on the campus. Seung-Hui Cho, a student at Virginia Tech majoring in English, was soon identified as the shooter who took his own life as law enforcement officials closed in on him at the end of his killing spree.

The tragedy ignited a debate on a number of fronts that are relevant to our discussion of therapeutic jurisprudence and school violence. Evidence collected after the shooting clearly indicated that Cho was suffering from significant psychological problems. Cho was originally described as a loner but evidence accumulated in the days after the incident that indicated his troubles ran much deeper. Several former professors commented that his class writings had been disturbing and at least one professor complained to administrators in her department. The University had investigated Cho for stalking two female students and in 2005 he was declared mentally ill, was hospitalized briefly, and was court ordered to seek outpatient therapy. However, Cho never followed the court's order and there was no follow-up of his case to determine if he had complied. Despite this court order questioning his mental soundness and a federal law prohibiting the sale, Cho was allowed to purchase the semi-automatic weapons he used in the shootings. The events leading up to the Virginia Teach tragedy and the deaths of over 30 people raise questions about the therapeutic interaction of the mental health and legal systems to prevent future incidents.

shooting of 10 girls ranging from 6 to 13 years-old at the West Nickel Mines Amish School in Pennsylvania in 2006. Of course, the horrific tragedy at Virginia Tech 2007 (Box 11.3) has become the most recent example and also serves as a reminder of the potential anti-therapeutic impact of our legal and mental health system. It is even more interesting that two of these last three examples of shootings bring attention to school violence when they were either not perpetrated by students, as in the case of West Nickel Mines Amish School, or juveniles were not the intended victims, as with Dawson College. Nonetheless, these sensationalized events add more fuel to the belief that school violence, specifically school shootings, is on the rise. Even at the height of the concern in the 1990s, school shootings did not sky rocket (Cornell, 2005) and even decreased following the 1997–8 school year (National School Safety Center, 2003; U.S. Surgeon General, 2001). In fact, violent crime in general has decreased in school (DeVoe et al., 2002). Schools continue to be one of the safest places for children (Shoemaker & Wolfe, 2005) and the probability of a student-perpetrated homicide occurring at school is .0000781 annually (Cornell, 2005).

Nonetheless, there has been greater attention placed upon school violence and forensic psychologists have been called to assist in the process. Early

Table 11.2.   Myths Surrounding School Shootings

School violence is an epidemic in the United States
School violence is increasing
Homicides are increasing in schools
All school shooters are alike
The school shooter is always a loner
School shootings are exclusively motivated out of revenge
Easy access to weapons is the most significant risk factor for school shootings
Students who become violent engage in a number of unusual hobbies and activities

Source: Based on O'Toole (2000) and Cornell (2007)

prevention efforts focused on zero tolerance policies and on identifying warning signs of possible school shooters. However, concerns arose that school administrators would use these lists of warning signs to identify and punish students. It should be noted that these lists of warning signs tended to include very general items such as previous truancy, use of drugs or alcohol, and frequent displays of anger. However, not even the most successful profilers in the world, the Federal Bureau of Investigation's (FBI) National Center for the Analysis of Violent Crime recommended profiling school shooters (O'Toole, 2000). The inappropriateness of the use of profiling is even more surprising given the so called "profiles" of school shooters that developed after incidents like Columbine. The public received the message that school shooters were all students who had been bullied and dressed in black trench coats. This view became so popular that the FBI identified a list of prominent myths (Table 11.2) that surrounded school shootings (O'Toole, 2000).

Although criminal profiling school shooters was not deemed an effective method for preventing them, the process of threat assessment that was mentioned before did seem to apply to these situations. Threat assessment was an approach developed by the United States Secret Service that was based on identifiable threats or attacks on public figures (Fein & Vossekuil, 1998, 1999). Threat assessment seems especially appropriate for school shooting because school shooters almost always tell someone about their plan beforehand and there is evidence that legitimate school shootings have been prevented because fellow students or adults have reported threats to authorities (O'Toole, 2000). Threat assessment does not cast a broad net over students like those warning lists did but instead assesses the viability of a threat because, as the FBI has suggested, not all threats are created equal and some will be completely harmless and others should be taken seriously (O'Toole, 2000). Threat assessment encourages identification of precise actions that are associated with behaving violently. For example, if a student makes a threat against a school and after an investigation it appears the student has access to weapons, has a specific plan, and has an identified target then the threat may be credible. However, if another student makes the same threat but has not exhibited any of these behaviors the threat may not be credible. Furthermore, preliminary research has supported the use of threat assessment in preventing school shootings (see Randazzo et al., 2006 for a review).

Even though it is a myth that school violence is an epidemic, all school shooters look alike, they are all loners, they all act completely out of revenge, and that they can be effectively profiled (O'Toole, 2000), homicides and violence do occur within the confines of our schools. The occurrence of even a single violent act, much less a homicide, should encourage decisive action on the part of administrators. Forensic psychologists can assist schools by educating them and performing threat assessments based on the empirical literature when appropriate.

Summary

The juvenile courts have a unique role in the legal system. Historically, they functioned as quasi-criminal courts where juveniles were not treated as harshly as adults for their delinquent behaviors but also were not afforded the same due process protections. This traditional approach to juvenile justice began to change in the United States in the 1960s because of perceptions that the rights of juveniles may be violated and that the juvenile court may not have fulfilled its original rehabilitative mission. These trends continued into the 1970s, as research concluded that "nothing works" in regard to juvenile rehabilitation and correctional treatment in general. The 1980s brought concern that juvenile violence was increasing astronomically and that we must treat juvenile crimes as we do adult criminal behavior. The publicity surrounding school shootings in the 1990s only heightened the public attention toward juvenile crime. However, the available empirical evidence suggests that juvenile crime, specifically juvenile violence is not currently on the rise. Nonetheless, we are left with a juvenile system that is more punitive in nature but continues to focus on the potential to rehabilitate. It is in the modern juvenile system that forensic psychology plays a more prominent role for better or worse. Even today, the juvenile courts are a much different system than our criminal courts. Processing in the juvenile courts consists of repeated attempts to identify the needs of the juvenile and to seek solutions outside of incarceration and detention.

The term juvenile delinquency is frequently used to describe the antisocial acts committed by juveniles that would normally be considered crimes if committed by an adult. However, juveniles may become involved in the juvenile court for a variety of other reasons such as for status offenses or as part of a child abuse or neglect investigation. In contrast to the public sentiment, juvenile crime and juvenile violence appear to be steadily decreasing, at least since the mid 1990s. Despite the widespread decrease in crime, there remain problematic issues. Juveniles account for a significant portion of criminal behavior and more juveniles are being sent to criminal courts to face adjudication and sentencing. Juvenile offenders also are becoming younger, female, and of minority status.

One positive outcome that may be related to the increased concern over juvenile delinquency is a greater awareness of the risk factors that lead to juvenile delinquency and juvenile violence. These risk factors are generally categorized into individual, family, peer, school, and neighborhood risk factors. Although there are unique factors for both delinquency and violence, there also appears to be some significant overlap in those factors that lead to both delinquency and violence and even lead to juveniles committing repeated delinquent and violent acts, or recidivating. In addition to identification of risk factors, there is increasing awareness of the protective factors, or factors that are likely to decrease juvenile offending. The resources devoted to sexual violence committed by juveniles has dramatically risen in the past 25 years, in part, because of the attention placed on juvenile crime but because of the public concern about sexual offending in general.

As public concern and governmental attention have grown, forensic psychologists have taken a more prominent role. Forensic psychologists continue to participate in their traditional roles by evaluating treatment amenability and offering psychological treatment. However, they also are increasingly stepping out of these traditional roles and evaluating juveniles for transfer to criminal court, conducting competency and insanity evaluations, and performing risk assessments. In addition, forensic psychologists are also performing a task directly related to the heightened media attention given to school shootings. Forensic psychologists are increasingly consulting with schools on ways to address school violence and prevent school shootings. A comparatively new approach borrowed from the Secret Service's attempts to prevent attacks on government officials is the use of threat assessments. Instead of profiling juveniles based on broad characteristics that may or may not be shared by the majority of school shooters, they examine juveniles who make threats and assess the credibility of those threats given the presence or absence of behaviors that are known to occur in youth who carry out those threats.

Key Terms

desistors	persistors	strength-based assessment
due process	status offense	threat assessment
juvenile delinquency		

Further Readings

Grisso, T., & Schwartz, R. G. (2000). *Youth on trial.* Chicago: University of Chicago Press.

Heilbrun, K., Goldstein, N. E. S., & Redding, R. E. (2005). *Juvenile delinquency: Prevention, assessment, and intervention.* New York: Oxford University Press.

12   Child Custody

This chapter continues to focus on child and family issues but in a different context than the previous two chapters by examining the legal and physical custody of children after their parents divorce or separate. Child custody may be one of the most difficult and complex issues in forensic psychology (Otto, Buffington-Vollum, & Edens, 2003) and it may be a personal and professional challenge to forensic psychologists because of the value-laden nature of these evaluations. In a child custody evaluation, a forensic psychologist must evaluate multiple people (parents, children, other potential caregivers); they must evaluate them in regard to numerous abilities and from multiple vantage points. The professional tasks become even more difficult with the added realization that child custody situations may pull on a professional's own personal biases in regard to raising children. Although any forensic task may pull on one's personal biases, many argue that child custody determinations are like no other forensic task in this regard. The value-laden nature of child custody evaluations becomes clearer when we think about our own ideas regarding the types of people who are the best parents or the manner in which we think children should be raised. Do you think two parents is the best way to raise a child? Are a man and a woman the best equipped to raise a child? Should children be spanked when they misbehave? Is a child better off with a parent of their own race or ethnicity? Is it better for a child to go to church, synagogue or temple or be raised by a parent who is not religious? These types of questions often address beliefs and values that everyone holds but may or may not be supported by the psychological literature. As a result, forensic psychologists who are involved in child custody decisions must be aware of their personal biases and acknowledge where their biases must end and their professional responsibilities begin. Furthermore, forensic psychologists may be less equipped and have less expertise in this area than other areas of forensic practice (Melton et al., 1997). All of these issues combine to make child custody situations extremely difficult and make it even more important that forensic psychologists are aware of practicing within their scope of practice.

It also is important to realize the frequency of these types of decisions before the courts today. It has been regularly discussed in the media that approximately half of all marriages end in divorce. However, not all married couples have children. Some research suggests that around 40% of children will experience the divorce of their parents prior to age 18 (Bumpass, 1984). Even more importantly, not all divorced couples with children will legally contest child custody. In fact, contesting the legal custody of children occurs in a minority of divorces. The best available data seem to suggest that only about 10–30% of cases involve legal conflict about the custody of children (Bernet, 2002; Maccoby, Mnookin, Depner, & Peters, 1992; McIntosh & Prinz, 1993).

Moreover, the courts may not accept expert testimony from forensic psychologists in the same manner in child custody decisions as they do in other cases. In previous chapters, there has been a general trend that the final decisions made by the courts are overwhelmingly similar to the conclusions reached by the consulting forensic psychologist. However, courts appear wearier of opinions offered by forensic psychologists in child custody decisions. Courts may be less likely to adopt the conclusions of forensic psychologists in this area than any other area in forensic psychology (Otto et al., 2003) and generally consider psychological evaluations less critical (Felner, Rowlison, Farber, Primavera, & Bishop, 1987). Horvath, Logan, and Walker (2002) found that the courts' ultimate decisions were identical to the conclusions of the child custody evaluation 27.3% of the time and similar in 63.6% of the cases. These numbers stand in stark contrast to the agreement rates we saw in earlier chapters focusing on insanity and competency decisions that were above 90%. Despite the courts' potential skepticism, it also appears that forensic psychologists are increasingly being retained in these cases (Emery, Otto, & O'Donohue, 2005).

Legal History and Assumptions About Child Custody

It is important to get a clear understanding of the meaning of custody before examining the legal assumptions involved. Traditionally, the law considered children **chattel**, or personal property, that must be divided when the marriage contract terminated or a divorce occurred. Common law originally considered children just like any other form of personal property but this practice has changed over the years so that there are now unique aspects in awarding custody of children, compared to other personal property like a couch or a fish tank.

There are several specific types of custody arrangements involving children (Hess, 2006). There is **sole custody** where one parent is awarded custody of the children. **Divided custody** occurs when each parent is awarded sole custody at different parts of the year. For example, a mother may be awarded sole custody of the child during the school year but then the child lives with the father during the summer. There is **split custody** where the custody of multiple children is split between two parents. For example, the mother may have sole custody of the daughter and the father may have sole custody of the son. Finally, there is **joint custody** where parents share custody of a child or children and both have ongoing responsibility for their care. Regardless of the specific type of custody, a parent also may have either legal or physical custody of a child. **Physical custody** means that the child lives with a particular parent and that parent is primarily responsible for the daily care of that child. **Legal custody** refers to the ability to make legal decisions regarding a child. So, a father may have sole physical custody of a child but the parents have joint legal custody so that both or either can make legal decisions regarding her care such as giving consent for a medical procedure. For simplicity, when we use the word custody, we are typically referring to physical custody or where the child lives.

Legal Standards and Preferences for Child Custody

The relevance of therapeutic jurisprudence is quite evident in some of the assumptions the law has made about who is the best parent. As previously stated, children have long been considered personal property and subject to division like any other personal property during a divorce. Originally, personal property reverted to the husband and therefore children also fell to the father (Wyer, Gaylord, & Grover, 1987). However, beginning in the late 1800s the law began to adopt a new preference in awarding the custody of children called the **tender years doctrine**.

Under the tender years doctrine the mother was considered the best parent, especially of children who were younger, or of tender years. The mother was considered inherently a better parent than the father because of her maternal and caring nature. Although mothers were typically considered the better qualified parents under the tender years doctrine, this legal preference could be overcome by showing the mother was unfit in some way and therefore should not receive custody of the children. This preference was adopted despite the fact that evidence clearly indicates that fathers can be as competent in their parenting as mothers (Silverstein, 1996). The tender years doctrine was the primary legal standard in most jurisdictions until about the 1970s (Hall, Pulver, & Cooley, 1996). At this time, the legal standard switched to the **best interest of the child**.

The adoption of this standard marked an important shift in the therapeutic intentions of the courts. The best interest of the child standard (BICS) suggests that the rights of the parents were not of primary importance in awarding custody of children but that the awarding of custody should be based on the development and continued maturation of the child. However, the best interest of the child standard is open to a great deal of interpretation and has been frequently criticized for its vagueness (Krauss & Sales, 2000). The Uniform Marriage and Divorce Act (1979) has been adopted by many jurisdictions and it considers a host of factors but without any specific weight. These factors include: (1) the mental and physical health of all individuals involved in the

Table 12.1.   Michigan's Best Interest of the Child Criteria

1. The love, affection, and other emotional ties existing between the parties involved and the child.
2. The capacity and disposition of the parties involved to give the child love, affection, and guidance and to continue the education and raising of the child in his or her religion or creed, if any.
3. The capacity and disposition of the parties involved to provide the child with food, clothing, medical care or other remedial care recognized and permitted under the laws of this state in place of medical care, and other material needs.
4. The length of time the child has lived in a stable, satisfactory environment, and the desirability of maintaining continuity.
5. The permanence, as a family unit, of the existing or proposed custodial home or homes.
6. The moral fitness of the parties involved.
7. The mental and physical health of the parties involved.
8. The home, school, and community record of the child.
9. The reasonable preference of the child, if the court considers the child to be of sufficient age to express preference.
10. The willingness and ability of each of the parties to facilitate and encourage a close and continuing parent-child relationship between the child and the other parent or the child and the parents.
11. Domestic violence, regardless of whether the violence was directed against or witnessed by the child.
12. Any other factor considered by the court to be relevant to a particular child custody dispute.

Source: Michigan Compiled Laws, 1970

care of the children; (2) the adjustment of the child to their home, school, and community; (3) parents' ability to provide basic needs; (4) interaction of the child with parents, siblings or any other individuals; (5) the wishes of the parents and the child; and (6) any other relevant factors. Michigan's Best Interest of the Child Criteria (1970) has also been frequently used as a model list of criteria (see Table 12.1).

Research has also asked child custody experts to rate the importance of these criteria in deciding custody arrangements based on the BICS. Results reveal that emotional ties between parents and child, willingness and ability of the parents to encourage a close parent–child relationship with the other parent, and the absence of domestic violence, were the most important to forensic psychologists in performing these evaluations (Bow & Quinnell, 2001). Moral fitness, home, school and community records of the child, and the permanence of the family unit were the least important (Bow & Quinnell, 2001). Although, the BICS may not offer definitive guidance as to the specific factors that should be considered and the weight that should be assigned to them, the standard does focus the attention back on the needs of the child, instead of the battling parties.

Additional Legal Preferences

Though rarely resulting in the development of precise legal standards, courts have also shown other preferences in awarding custody. There clearly has been a traditional preference for awarding custody to the biological parent or even biological relatives. This biological preference is clearest when the court has had to make decisions between a biological parent with a minimal or nonexistent relationship with the child and a third party with a significant interpersonal relationship with the child but no biological tie. This biological connection or blood tie has been so important in the eyes of the law that it extends even to fifth degree relatives anywhere from grand parents to great-great-great grandparents, uncles and aunts to great uncles and great aunts, and first cousins to first cousins once removed (Robbins, 1995). The courts have shown a resistance to awarding custody to non blood relatives, even when a prior relationship existed (*Bowie v. Arder*, 1991; Langelier & Nurcombe, 1985), because they assumed a biological relative is better qualified to raise a child than a non biological relative. This preference may even be based to some degree on the historical treatment of children as personal property.

In addition to the assumption that biological relatives are better qualified to raise a child, other legal assumptions have been challenged as society has evolved. The courts have assumed that in cases where there is a gay or lesbian parent that the heterosexual parent is more qualified to raise the child or the homosexual parent is even less qualified than another biological relative (*Bottoms v. Bottoms*, 1995). However, more recent trends suggest that some courts are ignoring the sexual orientation of any custodial parent as they appear to be unrelated to parenting ability (e.g., *Pulliam v. Smith*, 1998). Though the court specifically stated in *Pulliam* that homosexual parents receive equal consideration to heterosexual parents, the child in this case curiously was removed from the home of the homosexual parent because he was not married to his life partner and there were pictures of drag queens in the house.

Another issue the courts have addressed at times is awarding custody of children when the parents are of different races or then remarry someone of a different race. Originally, a child was placed with the parent he or she most physically resembled because the assumption was that the parent could best identify with any issues that child faced. The courts continue to struggle with this issue without a consistent trend. However, the United States Supreme Court has ruled that removing a child from a Caucasian mother because of her marriage to an African-American man is discriminatory (*Palmore v. Sidoti*, 1984). It is curious that the psychological literature did not support these legal assumptions and trends and any forensic psychologists who supported these legal realities with their testimony did so without clear empirical evidence.

Child Custody Laws and Professional Guidelines

As previously stated, the dominant legal standard today for awarding custody of a child is the best interest of the child standard. Hall et al. (1996) conducted a review of all the state statutes regarding custody determination and concluded that little consensus existed regarding the factors to be considered. They noted that the most commonly listed criteria include the child's wishes (24 of 50 states), observed interaction and interrelationship of the child, parents, and other parties (17 of 50), and history of child abuse (16 of 50). As of 2004, all states had adopted some form of the Uniform Child Custody Jurisdiction Act, similar to the Uniform Marriage and Divorce Act, that included several factors to be considered when determining the best interest of the child such as the age and sex of the child, the wishes of the child, interrelationship of the child, parents, siblings, and significant others, the child's adjustment to home, school and community, and the mental and physical health of all parties (Hess, 2006). Forensic psychologists must be aware of the precise laws in effect in their given jurisdiction regardless of any similarities or inconsistencies across different jurisdictions.

The BICS has been criticized for several reasons. First, critics have argued that there is no precise definition of the best interest of a child and therefore judicial decisions are often based on personal biases, not scientific literature or even societal notions (Schneider, 1991). It also has been argued that judges are not trained to make these determinations because they are based on a number of inexact non legal factors (Krauss & Sales, 2000). As a result, critics have argued that judges really use a default standard for making custody decisions, the least detrimental alternative standard (Schultz, Dixon, Lindberger, & Ruther, 1989). Scholars argue that judges use a negative standard by which the parent who is likely to cause the least amount of harm to the child is granted custody and that a formalization of this standard may provide the most useful standard (Krauss & Sales, 2000). This standard may be better because it more accurately represents the current practice of judges and societal expectations, it may be more realistic given some of the negative consequences of post-divorce relationships, psychological research is better at providing evidence of detrimental factors, and forensic evaluations based on this standard probably better represent the legitimate scope of practice of mental health professionals (Krauss & Sales, 2000). Although we will revisit some of these issues later, it is important to start thinking about the difficulties or the therapeutic consequences of the current BICS standard when the discussion turns to the practice of conducting child custody evaluations.

Professional Guidelines for Child Custody Evaluations

In addition to the legal standards that govern the parental preferences, there are a variety of professional guidelines that act as a guide for forensic psychologists

8. actively participates in child's education;
9. exhibits significant anger; and
10. bitterness about the divorce. (Ackerman & Ackerman, 1997)

Overall, it appears that child custody evaluations are becoming more comprehensive than in the past (Bow & Quinnell, 2001). Child custody evaluators are experienced, having on average 22 years of experience, 15 years in forensic practice, and 13 years in child custody evaluations (Bow & Quinnell, 2001). Furthermore, the overwhelming majority of child custody evaluators have experience with children, adolescents and adults (Bow & Quinnell, 2001). Forensic psychologists appear to be adhering to many of the professional recommendations. For example 99% of experts report informing participants of the limits of confidentiality, with 88% explaining it in written form. On the whole, these results suggest child custody evaluators are very qualified and diligent in their efforts.

Despite indications of overall competence in the field, there remains room for significant improvement. Horvath et al. (2002) took a different approach to much of the earlier research that asked child custody evaluations about their typical approaches to conducting child custody evaluations. Instead Horvath et al. (2002) examined the evaluations themselves. They found that in keeping with APA standards most psychologists used multiple methods for gathering information (84.3% at least two, 58.8% at least three, and 33.3% at least four). The majority of the evaluators assessed the psychological and developmental needs of the child (80.4%). Overall, results found that in practice there is considerable variation in the frequency in which critical factors are addressed in these evaluations and therefore some disagreement with previous research that asked for child custody experts about their routine practice. Horvath et al. suggest these differences may represent the differences between actual practice and the best practice standards experts are likely to admit to or encourage. Also, in contrast to previous research and scholarly opinion, Horvath et al. suggested that attorneys and judges are placing importance on the recommendations of the evaluations. In total, the results suggest there is still room for improvement in the routine practice of conducting child custody evaluations and that there should be continued evaluation and encouragement and education of the best practice standards. Overall though, it appears that forensic psychologists are doing a credible and increasingly better job in these difficult circumstances.

Difficulties in Child Custody Evaluations

It should already be clear from our prior discussion that child custody evaluations are some of the most difficult, if not the most difficult, evaluations undertaken by forensic psychologists for several reasons. It is one of the few forensic evaluations where the forensic psychologist must evaluate multiple people that are central to the legal question. This process is not a matter of only gathering collateral information from multiple sources and interviewing multiple people. This process should be a part of all or most forensic evaluations. In child custody evaluations the examiner is actually evaluating multiple people including potentially several children along with their parents and their parents' partners (Otto et al., 2003).

The breadth and depth of knowledge necessary for conducting child custody evaluations is significant. Someone who conducts child custody evaluations must be an expert not only in adult mental health but also childhood psychopathology, normal childhood development, and parenting practices. An evaluator must be skilled in a variety of assessment methods and be able to synthesize this information from multiple people in a clear and focused manner. Furthermore, forensic evaluators frequently suffer from a lack of empirical information in a number of different areas involving child custody evaluations (e.g., best custody arrangements for children) that make it even more difficult and raise the issue of the scope of practice limitations (Melton et al., 1997).

Not only is there a lack of empirical information regarding many of the areas involved in child custody evaluations but the standard psychological tests are often inadequate and forensic relevant instruments are no better at addressing the legal question. For example, it is not clear the extent to which psychopathology and intelligence are important constructs in determining child custody and their relationship to parenting skills. In fact, there appears to be a decrease in the prevalence of intelligence testing in these situations. Though there are a number of forensic relevant instruments for child custody evaluations, they have been routinely criticized as inappropriate, ill-conceived, or severely lacking in empirical support. However, this book highlighted similar criticisms about other areas of forensic practice (e.g., insanity) so it is unclear whether these instruments are inferior to efforts in other areas of forensic practice.

Another difficulty with conducting child custody evaluations is their value-laden nature. The nature of custody disputes leads to an evaluation of parenting practices and a suggestion, subtle or overt, as to the best parenting practices. An evaluator and the court are in a position to censure a parent for spanking their children, allowing them to stay up too late, allowing them to watch too much television or a host of other serious questions that parents routinely struggle with in raising children. A forensic psychologist may have a tendency to fall back on personal values and biases in determining a forensic opinion. A forensic psychologist should be aware of certain hot button issues such as domestic violence or infidelity. These issues may or may not be related to the forensic opinion but certainly should only be given the appropriate weight and not unduly influence the evaluator. The question remains though whether custody evaluations are all that unique in this concern.

Child custody evaluations tend to be extremely conflictual for the psychologist as well as the other parties involved. There are two parties that are obviously fighting over their child or children and divorces are frequently very emotional situations. In addition, a forensic psychologist may be the person whom one party or even both parties blame for an unfavorable custody arrangement. As a result, forensic psychologists who perform custody evaluations are frequent targets of ethical complaints and malpractice lawsuits (Benjamin & Gollan, 2003). Any psychologist thinking of practicing in this area should be aware that it is likely that they will be confronted with these situations.

The final difficulty that is a combination of many of the difficulties already discussed is the potential for child custody evaluations to fall outside the scope of practice of forensic psychologists. As discussed before, the legal standards for child custody evaluations are often criticized as problematic because they are frequently ambiguous or fall outside the expertise of psychology. Psychologists are not trained to determine the ability of parents to provide for the physical needs of children and many question the role that the psychological concepts that psychologists can assess (psychopathology and intelligence) should play in these evaluations. As a result, psychologists themselves have questioned whether forensic psychology has anything unique to offer the courts in these situations (Otto et al., 2003). Some have even argued that these situations fall outside the expertise of psychology because of the limitations of the research and the legal questions that are being asked.

Because of the difficulty both inherent in the custody evaluation process and the limitation of the relevant research, Emery et al. (2005) identified three reforms. First, they encouraged parents to reach agreements regarding child custody by other means than directly contesting it. Mediation, negotiation, therapy, and other means are encouraged prior to any adversarial approach. Mediation is described more fully later in this chapter. Second, they believe that legislatures should improve on the current standards for determining child custody by providing more definitive criteria that would even further narrow the practice scope. Emery et al.'s (2005) final recommendation is to limit expert testimony in the area. Limiting expert testimony can occur by forensic psychologists making a greater effort to only offer conclusions that are empirically based and to avoid moving beyond the available scientific literature, expanding professional guidelines, and utilizing the existing laws governing the admissibility of expert testimony. They go so far as to argue for a ban of any forensic relevant tests and argue for cautious use of general psychological tests applied to this area.

However, you should not get the idea from this chapter that child custody evaluations are without merit. Though the difficulties involved in conducting child custody evaluations may be significant, many of the criticisms of child custody evaluations are similar to the concerns raised about other areas of forensic practice. Even if you accept the criticisms fully, one question remains. Who would assist the court in deciding the best interest of the child if not mental health professionals? A plumber? As long as the courts are aware of the limitations of forensic practice in this area, which forensic psychologists should be making them aware of, the courts can assign the appropriate weight to the expert's reports and testimony in making their final legal decisions.

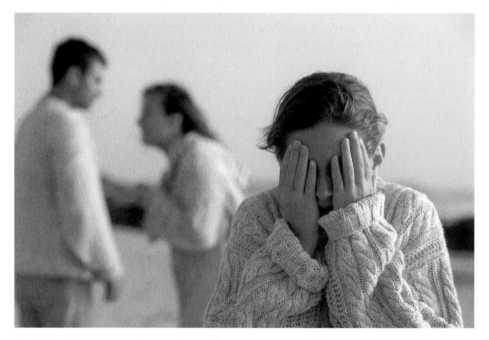

Figure 12.1. The marital conflict that often accompanies divorces and custody disputes can have a significant impact on the development of the children involved. ©
Getty Images/David De Lossy

Effects of Custody and Divorce on Children

In addition to the practice issues involved in child custody disputes, forensic
psychologists conducting these evaluations should also be aware of the impact
that divorce may have on children and the influence of different custody
arrangements (see Figure 12.1). There is a great deal of misinformation regarding the role of divorce and custody on the development of children. This misinformation may be the result of value-based judgments as well as early research
that had limited application because of methodological flaws. It is important
for any forensic psychologists to have a thorough understanding of these issues
when conducting custody evaluations.

Effects of Divorce on Children

Whether because of methodological limitations of the early research or the
social stigma attached to the divorce, initial research focusing on the developmental impact of divorce on children was fairly clear. The research consistently
suggested that children from divorced families suffered from a host of academic
and emotional difficulties that children from intact families did not experience
(Kelly, 2000). A more recent meta-analysis has suggested that these differences
only increase with age (Amato, 2001). Wallerstein and Blakeslee (1989)

Allegations of physical and sexual abuse may be becoming more prominent, though they still only occur in a minority of divorces, and forensic psychologists should be especially careful when a custody dispute involves abuse allegations.

Key Terms

best interest of the child	joint custody	sole custody
chattel	legal custody	split custody
divided custody	mediation	tender years doctrine
fact witness	physical custody	

Further Readings

Emery, R. E., Otto, R. K., & O'Donohue, W. T. (2005). A critical assessment of child custody evaluations. *Psychological Science, 6,* 1–29.

Otto, R. K., Buffington-Vollum, J. K., & Edens, J. F. (2003). Child custody evaluation. In A. M. Goldstein (Ed.), *Handbook of psychology: Vol. 11. Forensic psychology* (pp. 179–208). New York: John Wiley & Sons, Inc.

or expectations of an evaluator can increase the likelihood of a client reporting certain symptoms (Williams et al., 1999). As a result, forensic psychologists should be especially mindful of assessing for malingering when evaluating personal injury claims.

As mentioned in Chapter 2, there are several approaches to assessing for malingering beyond the clinical interview. One of the most frequently utilized measures in personal injury evaluations is the MMPI or MMPI-2 (Lees-Haley, 1992). In terms of scope of practice, the MMPI-2 is identified as acceptable to use in assessing malingering by more experts (92%) than any other measure and recommended by 64% of experts in cases where malingering is suspected, closely followed by the Structured Interview of Reported Symptoms (SIRS; 58%) that we discussed in Chapter 2 (Lally, 2003). In addition to the clinical scales assessing for a variety of mental illnesses, the MMPI-2 also contains several scales designed to assess for unusual response styles such as exaggeration and defensiveness.

Studies examining the effectiveness of these scales have taken some interesting approaches. Cramer (1995) asked college students to read information about specific mental illness (e.g., Depression and Paranoid Schizophrenia) and then take the MMPI-2. These students could produce more accurate results than students told to fake symptoms of the disorder without any additional information about the specific disorders. However, Cramer (1995) could tell the informed fakers and the uninformed fakers from individuals actually suffering from the Depression and Paranoid Schizophrenia. These results have been replicated for other disorders and when financial incentives were offered to produce valid results for these disorders, as many as 95% of the malingerers were detected (Wetter, Baer, Berry, Robison, & Sumpter, 1993). Research also has suggested that several MMPI-2 scales may be able to identify individuals who attempt to fake head injuries (Berry & Butcher, 1998). MMPI-2 results for individuals involved in litigation are generally more exaggerated and suggest more mental illness than individuals not involved in litigation. However, these scales are not without limitations and forensic psychologists need to be aware of them when conducting personal injury evaluations (Butcher & Miller, 2006).

Typical Injuries Involved in Personal Injury Claims

There are a variety of different injuries exhibited by personal injury claimants that forensic psychologists may evaluate. This section will discuss three of the most prominent: posttraumatic stress disorder (PTSD), neuropsychological damage, and chronic pain. However, there are a variety of different psychologically related illnesses that someone may suffer in these situations. Generally, there are three broad areas of injuries that the courts will compensate plaintiffs for under tort law. Historically, courts were first likely to compensate victims who suffered physical injuries that led to psychological injuries. Courts probably had the easiest time compensating victims in these types of cases because the causal path was easily identified and seemed more legitimate in the eyes of the courts because the physical injury legitimized the psychological injury (Melton et al., 1997). An example of this type of injury would be if someone were mugged and in the process sustained a head injury. The head injury may lead to poor attention, a lack of concentration, some memory impairment, or even personality change.

Cases in which an individual suffers only a psychological injury are much more difficult. Although these instances have become much more common, being compensated for strictly psychological injuries is difficult (McLearen et al., 2003). The courts are more suspicious of these types of injuries because they believe there is often a lack of concrete evidence for the injury, compared to a physical injury. One of the earliest cases in which psychological injuries were seen as compensable occurred in 1348. In this case, a guest at an inn threw a hatchet at the innkeeper's wife but she avoided it and did not suffer any physical injuries. The innkeeper brought suit for mental pain and suffering and was awarded damages for his wife (Mendelson, 1995). Though strict psychological injury claims are difficult to prove in court, PTSD is becoming a common basis for injury in these cases, as we will discuss later in this chapter.

The third and final general type of injury that is compensable is the worsening of a preexisting psychological condition. A person with preexisting episodes of major depression could claim that the mugging she suffered increased the severity of the disorder and caused her to seek additional treatment. In these instances, it is important to have a clear idea of the person's baseline or premorbid functioning prior to the incident and an identified period of stability. The difficulties involved in these types of cases should be clear. Not only does the plaintiff have to prove the existence of a psychological illness or injury but the plaintiff must prove that it has become worse since the specific event in question.

Posttraumatic Stress Disorder (PTSD)

PTSD probably represents the single largest psychological disorder for plaintiffs in personal injury cases and may have a greater impact on the court system than any other mental illness in history (Stone, 1993). As suggested before, there is probably a reason for the increasing reliance on PTSD in personal injury litigation. PTSD provides a way for a plaintiff to make her emotional suffering more tangible by having it supported by the presence of a psychological disorder. However, major depression and many other anxiety disorders also provide more tangible anchors than general emotional pain and suffering. Is there something else about PTSD? Yes, PTSD is the only mental illness that, as part of its diagnostic criteria, necessitates a specific triggering event for the disorder to be diagnosed. This causal relationship, whether any different than most psychological disorders or not in reality, provides a more clear causal relationship for the courts. Given that a specific event must be the proximate cause of the psychological injuries, the courts look favorably on this type of causal pathway.

In addition to the presence of a traumatic event, referred to as Criterion A (i.e., presence of a trauma) in the diagnostic criteria of DSM, there are three additional major symptom groups for PTSD (APA, 2000). In order to be diagnosed with PTSD a person must present symptoms from Criteria A, B, C, and D for at least a month. If symptoms are present for two days to four weeks, the person can be diagnosed with another mental illness, Acute Stress Disorder. Criterion B consists of different reexperiencing symptoms such as upsetting memories of the event, distressing dreams, and flashbacks. Criterion C is the avoidance cluster of symptoms and includes symptoms like trying to avoid thoughts, feelings, places, or people associated with the trauma and the inability to recall certain important information about the trauma. The final group of symptoms, Criterion D, focuses on increased arousal such as sleep disturbances, a heightened startle response, or excessive vigilance to the surrounding environment. Depending on the group of symptoms, a person must experience a traumatic event meeting Criterion A, and experience, one, three, or two symptoms from Criteria B, C, and D respectively.

Experiencing many of these symptoms is quite normal for someone who has experienced a traumatic or extremely anxiety provoking situation. For example, many people are involved in a car accident at some point in their lifetime. If you or someone you know was, did you experience any of these symptoms afterward? Did you avoid driving after the accident? Were you extra cautious or vigilant when you were driving, stopping at stop signs, or crossing intersections? Were you startled when you heard some tires screeching? Although these types of reactions are quite normal after a car accident, to be diagnosed with PTSD a particular number of these symptoms must last for one month and are considered chronic PTSD if they last for at least 3 months (APA, 2000).

The only problem from a legal standpoint is that PTSD is increasingly seen as having multiple causes. Originally, it was believed that people would develop PTSD as a result of exposure to a traumatic event, originally deemed to be "outside the normal range of human experience" when first identified in DSM-III (APA, 1980, p. 238). Now the event must "involve intense fear, helplessness, or horror" and the person must be "confronted with an event or events that involved actual or threatened death or serious injury, or a threat to the physical integrity of self or others" (APA, 2000, p. 467). It was the exposure to the traumatic event that was believed to be the cause or the single most important cause of PTSD.

Evolving research has now suggested that there are a range of factors outside of the original trauma including events pre trauma and post trauma that contribute to the development of PTSD (Young & Yehuda, 2005). Factors prior to the trauma such as a history of other mental illness, and particular personality patterns related to negative emotion or excessive anxiety (Blanchard et al., 1996;

Mason, Turpin, Woods, Wardope, & Rowlands, 2006) increase the likelihood that someone exposed to a traumatic event will develop PTSD. Other post trauma factors such as fear of dying in the situation, additional psychosocial stressors, loss of social support, the pursuit of litigation, and presence of appropriate therapy relate to the development of PTSD (Blanchard et al., 1996; Mason et al., 2006; Young & Yehuda, 2005). Most people who actually experience a traumatic event that would qualify under Criterion A, maybe almost as many as 70%, do not develop PTSD. This multicausal conceptualization of PTSD may limit its future use in court or open it up to criticism in a legal context. Courts believe that a forensic psychologist can easily differentiate the factors that occurred before the trauma, from the trauma and the events that occurred after the trauma but this process often proves extremely difficult (Young & Yehuda, 2005). However, in the future courts may find the evolving research supporting neurobiological markers and characteristic physiological responses for individuals with PTSD as more tangible for legal purposes and once again make PTSD a more acceptable justification for emotional pain and suffering from a legal perspective (Mendelson, 1995).

Forensic psychologists assessing PTSD in personal injury cases have a variety of established measures at their disposal but should be cautious assessing PTSD in the litigation context. The current gold standard for the assessment of PTSD may be the Clinician Administered PTSD Scale (CAPS) and research indicates that it is a reliable and valid tool for the assessment of PTSD (Koch, O'Neil, & Douglas, 2005). In addition to assessing the specific symptoms in Criteria B, C, and D, a forensic psychologist must establish that the trauma meets Criterion A. Currently, there is no psychological measure that can definitively assess whether PTSD was caused by a specific legal claim (Greenberg, Otto, & Long, 2003). A forensic psychologist can therefore either take an objective approach and focus on the severity of the physical injury or the resulting personal property damage (Malmquist, 1996) or undertake a more comprehensive view that may include some subjective indications (Koch et al., 2005).

However, courts may be weary of considering the client's subjective responses even though it does not appear to increase the prevalence of PTSD dramatically (see Koch et al., 2005). In addition, assessments of PTSD Criterion A require a thorough examination of past traumatic events, which increases the likelihood of suffering from PTSD. Given that the majority of people experience a traumatic event in their lifetime, it is important for the examiner to also screen for past trauma exposure in order to meet tort elements. Plaintiffs suffering from PTSD also are more likely to recall more symptoms than originally reported. Harvey and Bryant (2000) interviewed accident victims one month and two years after their accidents. Individuals who were experiencing more severe PTSD symptoms after two years recalled suffering from more symptoms two years later than they originally recalled at one month post accident. Individuals experiencing no symptoms two years post accident actually now under reported the trauma symptoms they originally reported at one month.

Traumatic Brain Injury (TBI)

In addition to PTSD, a significant number of personal injury litigants may suffer from a head injury or traumatic brain injury (TBI). The growth of these types of evaluations is clear by noting that prior to 1980, neuropsychologists were rarely ever involved in the legal system but today most neuropsychologists are involved in forensic assessments because of their evaluation of individuals presenting with TBIs (Barth, Ruff, Espe-Pfeifer, 2005; Taylor, 1999). The severity of a TBI is usually associated with the length of time the person is unconscious, the extensiveness of any associated amnesia, and the presence of a penetrating injury to the skull. Mild TBIs are usually characterized by less than 30 minutes of unconsciousness and a lack of serious injury to the exterior of the skull. The Glasgow Coma Scale (GCS) is an observational scale used as a brief assessment of head injuries. The scale is used to assess general consciousness and involves an assessment of the injury victim's motor and verbal abilities with scores ranging from three to fifteen. Scores of three to eight indicate a severe TBI, nine to twelve indicate a moderate TBI and thirteen to fifteen indicate a mild TBI (Barth et al., 2005). However, there is confusion and disagreement about specific definitions for different severity levels of TBIs that can make diagnosis difficult (Barth et al.).

The Centers for Disease Control and Prevention estimate that 1.5 million people annually suffer from TBIs and that 75% of these people suffer mild TBIs (mTBI) in a variety of different ways (as cited in Barth et al., 2005). The most common cause of mTBIs are motor vehicle accidents (42%), falls (24%), assaults with a firearm (14%) and concussions due to sports related activities (12%) (Parker, 2001) (see Figure 13.1). However, only a minority of victims (15%) continue to experience symptoms for longer than one year (Guerrero, Thurman, & Sniezek, 2000).

Neuropsychological evaluations of TBIs present many difficult tasks. It is difficult to assess premorbid level of functioning in neuropsychology cases, outside of prior testing. Courts commonly rely on forensic psychologists practicing neuropsychology to apply their test results to the real world, especially in regard to future functioning. This task can prove difficult because the examiner must generalize from the results of tests administered under very precise and constant conditions to real world environments that are anything but constant and controlled (McLearen et al., 2003). For example, I once had a client who did not exhibit any significant memory deficits on a host of neuropsychological measures. This same client would genuinely have difficulty finding her way home and had forgotten her son on top of her car, only to realize it when her husband came home later and noticed the infant in his car seat on top of the car. Finally, as with other injuries in personal injury cases, it is often very difficult to differentiate brain injuries from attempts to fake or feign the condition, especially when the TBI is fairly minor (Ackerman, 1999). Compound this general trend with the fact that it is not unusual to identify neuropsychological damage, even in individuals who are malingering or for normals trying

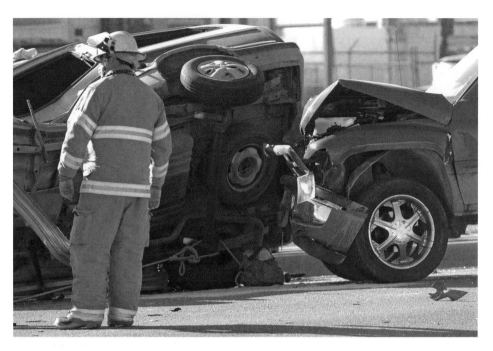

Figure 13.1. Motor vehicle accidents are a significant source of personal injury claims and the most prevalent cause of PTSD and mild TBIs. Photo © Lane V. Erickson/ Shutterstock

to look identical to brain injured individuals (Millis & Putnam, 1996). One survey of neuropsychologists revealed that they found indications of malingering in 29% of their personal injury referrals and that an identical percentage of individuals claiming mild head injuries exhibited indications of probable malingering (Mittenberg, Patton, Canyock, & Condit, 2002).

Despite their "objectivity" as a physically based injury and continued admissibility in courts (Stern, 2001, p. 93), forensic psychologists assessing neuropsychological disorders must go to great effort to assess for malingering in all aspects of their evaluation. Intelligence tests are commonly used in these assessments. In fact, Lees-Haley, Smith, Williams, and Dunn (1996) found that neuropsychologists used them in 76% of all their forensic evaluations. Fortunately, it is relatively difficult to malinger on intelligence tests without being detected. Attempted malingers normally provide inconsistent responses on the different subscales and are unsophisticated in many of their responses (Ackerman, 1999). Memory tasks are slightly different in that it is relatively easy for plaintiffs to malinger impairment on these tasks such as the Wechsler Memory Scale (WMS) and the Wechsler Memory Scale-Revised (WMS-R) but there are certain indications that differentiate malingerers from genuinely brain injured plaintiffs (Mittenberg, Tremont, & Rayls, 1996). There are also specifically designed tests to assess malingering in neuropsychological evaluations such as Rey's 15-item Visual Memory Test for the Detection of Malingering and the

Test of Memory Malingering (TOMM). In addition, many neuropsychological tests are forced choice tests where even chance responding would result in 50% correct, while malingerers frequently fall below chance in an attempt to look impaired.

There is significant controversy in the field of neuropsychology that directly impacts forensic practice. In general, there are two broad approaches to neuropsychological assessment. A neuropsychologist may either take the **fixed battery approach** or the **flexible process approach**. The fixed battery approach necessitates that the examiner administer a standardized set of neuropsychological tests in an identical manner to gain a comprehensive picture of the client. The fixed battery approach may sometimes mean that some of the tests are not directly relevant to the potential impairment and therefore administration time can be extensive. The fixed battery approach is the more traditional approach to administer neuropsychological tests and much of the empirical support behind different neuropsychological tasks is based on this approach. In the flexible process approach, an examiner is more selective about the specific tasks she asks of the examinee and usually selects tests that assess only those areas for which the symptoms suggest possible impairment. This approach is more directed and generally takes less time to administer. The controversy arises because many of the neuropsychological tests have not been empirically tested outside of their original battery and the examiner may miss indications of impairment that do not fall within their more limited parameters, as created by the selected number of tests. A legal issue arises because the flexible approach has been criticized, at times successfully, for not fulfilling the scientific admissibility criteria of *Daubert* (Chapter 3) or even just the general acceptance criteria. However, there also are instances in which the flexible battery approach has been admitted because it was generally accepted or met the *Daubert* requirements. The results of Lees-Haley et al. (1996) research seem to suggest that both approaches are generally widespread among neuropsychologists in forensic evaluations.

Chronic Pain

The final area in which personal injury claims and forensic psychology overlap is with the assessment of chronic pain. At first glance, it may seem that forensic psychologists would not have anything to do with evaluating someone for the degree of pain he is experiencing. Many people associate pain with a clear physical basis and assume that a physician would be solely responsible for assessing a patient's pain. However, the overwhelming majority of the time there is no objective test for the severity of pain a person is experiencing. Furthermore, pain is very much a psychological experience with people experiencing it differently depending on a host of psychological variables, despite similar physical injuries.

There is an extensive history examining the role of psychological factors in the subjective experience of pain (Gatchel & Kishino, 2005). There are long established correlations between personality and pain. Individuals who suffer from chronic pain are at greater risk for suicide, depression, anxiety, substance abuse (Dersh, Polatin, & Gatchel, 2002) and have been identified as one of the top health concerns by the Surgeon General (Hanscom & Jex, 2001). The belief of a specific personality type that is more susceptible to report chronic pain is largely outdated (Gatchel & Kishino, 2005). Though personality disorders are more common in chronic pain sufferers, there is little consistency regarding the specific personality disorder that is more likely in individuals who experience chronic pain (Gatchel & Kishino, 2005). Research also suggests there are a variety of cognitive factors that relate to the reporting of pain (Pincus, 2005). There appears to be good support for the role of locus of control, cognitive distortions such as catastrophizing, attention, avoidance of fear, and overall coping strategies in the pain experience (Linton, Vlaeyen, & Ostelo, 2002). For example, professionals have begun to recognize a difference between people who exhibit an active coping response and people who exhibit a passive coping response. Individuals who cope passively report greater pain (Pincus, 2005). Finally, return to work is often used as a sort of gold standard in chronic pain cases. Research suggests that psychosocial variables account for more of the reason for an individual returning to work than do physical symptoms (Gallagher et al., 1989).

The role of the forensic psychologist in regard to assessing and treating chronic pain is a difficult one. The forensic psychologist must be aware of the different psychological variables related to chronic pain but also be aware they may contribute to the pain experience or be a result of the person experiencing severe and chronic pain. For example, an individual may be more prone to experiencing chronic pain because of a personality style or may develop a certain personality style (e.g., depression) because the person has to live with a chronic disability. Gatchel and Weisberg (2000) recommend a stepwise approach in the assessment of chronic pain whereby clinicians begin with a global examination of the individual and progressively become more specific in the psychological factor they are assessing. Although there are a variety of personality measures such as the MMPI-2, Beck Depression Inventory, or the Symptom Checklist-90-Revised that are very appropriate for assessing personality in chronic pain patients, there are very few standardized measures for assessing the relevant cognitive factors (Pincus, 2005). Nonetheless, these data continue to be used to determine the person's potential for rehabilitation, which would factor directly into any compensation being sought (for example, lost wages, cost of therapy) and the extensiveness of any pain and suffering.

In addition to assessing for the psychological and cognitive dimensions that may be related to the pain experience, forensic psychologists should also assess for motivation (Gatchel & Kishino, 2005). People experiencing chronic pain often limit their activity to avoid experiencing the pain. People who become satisfied with these limitations after all medical options have been exhausted are poor candidates for a pain management program that can assist them in overcoming the limitations they may associate with their pain (Gatchel & Kishino,

2005). Besides general motivation to cope with the pain, there may be additional secondary gains associated with maintenance of the pain experience.

As with TBIs, there is evidence of a link between compensation for chronic pain and reports of chronic pain. A meta-analysis of the available studies focusing on chronic pain indicated that individuals who seek compensation report greater pain and are less likely to benefit from treatment (Rohling et al., 1995). Moreover, there has been a dramatic increase in the number of individuals seeking compensation for chronic pain. One study found almost a 2,700% increase in financial expenditures related to one chronic pain injury, lower back injuries, while the incidence of lower back pain remained constant (Fordyce, 1985). In fact, only one-quarter of all disability claims involve lower back pain but they still account for a majority of the compensation doled out for disability claims (Spengler et al., 1986).

As a result, it is extremely important to assess for malingering in chronic pain evaluations. Although there are measures to assess perceptions of chronic pain directly, many forensic psychologists assess the accompanying personality characteristics or additional neuropsychological symptoms for malingering. The MMPI-2 continues to be one of the more common methods used to assess malingering as well as be incorporated into chronic pain evaluations. There appear to be consistent differences on the MMPI-2 between individuals who are experiencing chronic pain and are seeking financial compensation and those who are not seeking compensation. Dush, Simons, Platt, Nation, and Ayres (1994) found that individuals seeking compensation through the courts were more likely to endorse obvious symptoms and less likely to endorse positive symptoms on the MMPI-2. In another study assessing neuropsychological symptoms among individuals with chronic pain, 29% of the individuals seeking compensation failed two or more validity checks in a series of neuropsychological tests, whereas none of the individuals failing to seek compensation failed two or more of those same validity checks (Meyers & Diep, 2000). Failing the validity checks on an instrument like the MMPI-2 suggests the person is giving distorted responses or potentially malingering. Forensic psychologists evaluating individuals who suffer from chronic pain therefore must be aware of the different response styles to personality and neuropsychological measures and the increased likelihood of malingering in these situations.

Psychological Independent Medical Evaluation

Although the majority of the chapter so far has focused on issues related to personal injury claims generally, there are also specific types of forensic assessments that occur in the civil context. Independent Medical Evaluations (IMEs) are evaluations that take place at the request of insurance companies in ongoing disability claims. Insurance companies may insure a particular individual and need an independent evaluation of the person's disability that prevents the person from working. These evaluations are very similar to personal injury evaluations except that they do not necessitate an evaluation of proximate cause. Although it may be appropriate to examine the underlying cause and circumstances, the forensic psychologist does not need to form an opinion as to whether the original circumstances were the proximate cause of any disability. Instead the forensic psychologist only needs to assess the ongoing symptoms and treatment effectiveness in relation to the person's ability to function in his or her place of employment (Vore, 2007).

Though psychological IMEs are similar to personal injury evaluations, there are significant differences from a legal standpoint. A basic issue in psychological IMEs is the definition of a disability that is preventing the person from working. A disability can be factual, social, or legal. A **factual disability** meets the criteria for a disability as stated in the insurance contract such as an illness or injury that prevents a person from carrying out their job or any job. A **social disability** usually refers to something which is not covered by the specific language of a contract. For example, a physician may contract a communicable disease that prevents her from performing as a surgeon. A **legal disability** usually refers to someone who is unable to work because of a license revocation or suspension. In general, these disability claims may relate to a specific occupation or any occupation and present an important consideration for a forensic examiner. The referral question may be whether the insured person is unable to work in their particular occupation because of a psychological injury or unable to work in any occupation. For example, it would be understandable if a lion tamer in a circus was unable to continue his job as a lion tamer after he was mauled by a lion. If his policy provided for compensation while he was unable to continue in his specific occupation, then he may be eligible for continued benefits. However, if the policy required that he be unable to perform in any occupation, the forensic psychologist would have to consider whether a particular psychological injury prevented him from working with the monkeys, operating a cotton candy machine or doing something totally unrelated to circus performing.

Overall, many of the same legal and clinical practice issues pertinent to forensic work in general pertain to psychological IMEs. Vore (2007) suggests that forensic psychologists performing psychological IMEs should follow the factors relevant to any forensic evaluation. These steps include conducting a thorough evaluation, identification of any specific deficits that would impair the ability of the insured to perform their job (not assessment of the legal issues related to the presence of a disability), base any opinion on clearly delineated objective data, and finally assess for the presence of distortion or malingering. As with all personal injury related claims, malingering or exaggeration is an especially important consideration (Richman et al., 2006). Forensic psychologists conducting psychological IMEs also should be mindful of additional legal and ethical issues relevant to forensic evaluations such as avoidance of dual relationships, identification of the client (i.e., the insurance company), informed consent, and scope of practice issues (Evans, 1992). In these instances, the law is increasingly scrutinizing the independent nature of these evaluations in order to avoid conflicts of interest that may arise from psychologists attempting to appear independent but actually working as default representatives of the insurance companies. Their intent was to provide a more therapeutic outcome by providing truly independent examinations.

Workers' Compensation

Another area of forensic practice that is related to personal injury is workers' compensation. Workers' compensation laws were intended to compensate employees who have been injured while performing work-related responsibilities. Employers purchase insurance to provide this benefit and employers are compensated for their injuries, regardless of whether the employee or the employer is at fault (Charlton, Fowler, & Ivandick, 2006). Before workers' compensation laws, employees who were injured on the job could only be compensated via personal injury claims as a matter of tort law. As a result, employers had a number of potential legal defenses in line with the tort law previously discussed (Melton et al., 1997). Workers' compensation laws were developed to reduce the difficulty employees had in receiving compensation for viable injuries suffered on the job because many saw the past system as a failure or anti-therapeutic.

However, in streamlining the personal injury process both parties relinquished certain legal rights they normally held. Employers cannot present many of the legal defenses that would have been available to them under tort law. The employees are not able to pursue the unlimited compensation that may arise from a personal injury lawsuit. Though the employers and employees must relinquish certain rights, the process has had an overall therapeutic impact (Lippel, 1999). Employees gave up the right for potentially unlimited compensation and instead received a greater likelihood of compensation and a fixed plan of compensation. Another interesting aspect of workers' compensation claims is that they are not designed to make the employee whole as are traditional compensatory damages in civil law. Workers' compensation is intended to replace lost earnings and pay for any additional expenses that may be incurred as a result of the work-related injury.

For the forensic psychologist, the process does not change a great deal. Employees seeking workers' compensation can suffer any of the same injuries suffered under personal injury claims. An employee could be making a delivery and be involved in an automobile accident in the course of that delivery. He may then develop PTSD (see Box 13.2 for a current issue in the assessment of work related PTSD) as a result and seek compensation through the workers' compensation program. Another employee working in a warehouse may suffer a lower back injury or fall while stacking material on a shelf and thereby suffer a head injury. In all of these cases, the employee can seek compensation through workers' compensation claims as they would have through a much more time consuming and uncertain personal injury claim. As long as these events result

Box 13.2.   The Role of Psychological Evaluations in Iraq War Combat Veterans

Although it does not fall under the umbrella of worker's compensation, the increasing prevalence of PTSD among veterans of the War in Iraq is related to our discussion of these claims. However, instead of falling under worker's compensation, veterans claiming PTSD are seeking to access disability benefits provided through their military benefits and military regulations. Moreover, these evaluations and the reception of these benefits are receiving increasing attention as veterans return from Iraq with rates of combat-related PTSD that may be two, three, or four times greater than previous combatants and with as many as 50% of those returning suffering from PTSD symptoms. Although these claims are not routinely handled as worker's compensation claims, they do involve the veteran's psychological evaluations to apply for disability benefits through the military. These disability evaluations resemble the forensic evaluations discussed in this chapter and are similar to another type of forensic evaluation not discussed in this chapter, evaluations for social security benefits. For example, they have specific requirements to meet much like the legal requirements for other civil issues. Military regulations require that the PTSD must not be the result of a preexisting condition, it must have been caused by their experiences while in the military, and the PTSD must result in a disability that prevents future service or reduces their ability to work in a civilian occupation. Furthermore, these situations are making headlines as at least one lawsuit has been filed against the Veterans Administration (VA) on behalf of the returning veterans that alleges the VA has failed to give mandatory disability benefits, address staff problems, and has provided insufficient care for veterans returning with posttraumatic stress disorder.

in an injury or disability, occur during the course of employment, and are accidental then workers' compensation laws are likely in effect (Meriano, 2001). As with all evaluations in which the examinee is seeking financial incentives, the forensic psychologist should make special efforts to assess for malingering or exaggeration of any symptoms in an attempt to receive greater compensation.

Sexual Harassment and Employment Discrimination

A final area of civil law that departs significantly from our previous discussion of traditional personal injury claims is the evaluation of sexual harassment and employment discrimination. Discrimination occurs in the workplace for a variety of reasons and the Civil Rights Act of 1964 identified gender, race, religion and national origin as protected classes of people who are legally protected against discrimination. Additional laws have provided protection for other groups of people and other specific legal mechanisms that may need to be addressed in addition to the requirements in the Civil Rights Action of 1964 (Vasquez, Baker, & Shullman, 2003). Furthermore, discrimination and harassment are not a completely independent entity and may arise in the context of workers' compensation and personal injury claims in general.

Discrimination claims either result from discriminatory effects or discriminatory treatment. **Discriminatory effects** require that the plaintiff show an entire group has been negatively impacted by a workplace policy or general practice. **Discriminatory treatment** only requires showing that one person has been harmed. Harassment is a form of discrimination that requires the workplace to have been adversely altered. Sexual harassment is a form of harassment that involves unwanted sexual behaviors. Research has found that roughly 49% of women and 33% of men received some type of unwanted sexual attention (see Douglas & Koch, 2001b). Sexual harassment can include **quid pro quo harassment** in which an employer or supervisor expects the employee to comply with sexual demands or behaviors in order to maintain his or her employment. It can also include hostile work harassment. **Hostile work harassment** applies to cases in which sexual demands or behaviors make the work environment unbearable (Douglas & Koch, 2001b).

The role of a forensic psychologist in discrimination and harassment claims is unique compared to the other areas explored in this chapter. The forensic psychologist is asked to determine whether the harassment or discrimination occurred, why it occurred, and the effects on the defendant (Vasquez et al., 2003). Of course, it is not within the scope of practice of a forensic psychologist to actually determine the physical occurrence of the discrimination or harassment or why it occurred. However, the forensic psychologist can examine the psychological state of the defendant after the alleged events to determine whether there is any support for the damage the defendant claims. There is also a significant social science literature examining the impact of discrimination and harassment in the workplace that any clinically trained forensic psychologist must consult (Fiske, 1998). For example, a forensic psychologist often must address whether the behavior was unwanted in determining why it occurred. The forensic psychologist should be aware that there is a significant difference in the way men and women generally perceive attention to be unwanted. It is incumbent on the forensic psychologist to be familiar with the psychological literature examining the myriad of individual differences and the impact of various forms of discrimination and harassment. This expertise is usually a new challenge for most forensic psychologists and should not be underestimated when considering whether one is qualified to conduct these types of evaluations. In addition to the unique legal requirements and the accompanying scientific literature, these evaluations involve the same content and procedures discussed throughout this text and this chapter. The examining forensic psychologist should be aware of the general legal difficulties such as identification of the client, the psychological tests that are appropriate and standardized in these situations, and the increased chance of malingering when financial incentives are at issue.

Summary

This chapter was devoted entirely to areas of civil law that are often ignored in discussions of forensic psychology. Personal injury and discrimination are based on tort law and present a host of challenges to forensic psychologists practicing in the area. Although forensic psychologists should stay within their scope of practice, it continues to be important for them to be familiar with the law governing torts and the more unique requirements specific to some of the specialized areas such as sexual harassment.

Tort law represents the legal framework for much of civil law and requires the presence of four elements to support a civil claim. There must be a duty that the defendant owed the plaintiff. There must have been some violation of that duty by the defendant. Damages must have occurred because of the violation of that duty. Finally, the violation of that duty must have been the proximate cause of the damages the plaintiff suffered. In traditional tort claims, all of these elements must be present for the plaintiff to pursue a lawsuit or receive damages from the defendant. Damages may be compensatory, meant to compensate the plaintiff, or punitive, meant to punish the defendant for the violation of the duty.

Although many of the previous forensic assessment issues pertain to personal injury cases, there are also somewhat unique tasks that the forensic psychologist must address. The forensic psychologist must establish a premorbid level of functioning to compare the current psychological state to determine the onset or worsening of any psychological injuries. The extent of the impairment that resulted from the injuries must be determined and the cause of the impairment must be determined. The final task is for the forensic psychologist to identify any interventions that will assist in reducing the injury or the impairment resulting from the injury.

An issue that appears to be especially important in personal injury cases is the likelihood of malingering or exaggeration of symptoms in order to receive additional financial considerations. There is clear evidence that individuals involved in a variety of different personal injury claims report more severe symptoms than originally reported prior to litigation and report more symptoms compared to injured individuals who do not pursue litigation. It is also clear that attorneys encourage clients to alter the responses they give to psychological and neuropsychological tests. This practice, while it may be legally ethical, compromises the psychological evaluation and presents a challenge to the forensic psychologist seeking to maintain the integrity of the assessment. There are a number of methods designed to assess for malingering and exaggeration including use of specially designed tools and built in validity scales for the most commonly used tests in these situations.

Personal injury lawsuits involve a variety of different injuries that may be evaluated by examining forensic psychologists. PTSD is psychological disorder that is especially geared toward use in civil law because of its unique diagnostic criteria. In order to be diagnosed with PTSD a person must be exposed to a

correctional psychology – branch of clinical psychology that focuses on the application of clinical psychology to individuals incarcerated in jails and prisons.

criminal law – law that focuses on disputes between individuals and society in general. The state or government is the representative of society in criminal law and brings charges against an individual for violating it.

criminal profiling – the process by which characteristics of a crime and crime scene are collected and systematically organized to narrow down the potential suspects.

Criminogenic needs – the goals that offenders have or the needs they fulfill when committing crimes.

deinstitutionalization – a process involving release of the mentally ill from psychiatric facilities and encouraging them to integrate into the community.

desistors – individuals who have committed juvenile crimes but discontinued their criminal pattern as adults.

diminished capacity – a legal defense that reduces or eliminates the criminal responsibility of a defendant because of a diminished mental state when a particular mental state is required for commission of a crime.

discriminatory effects – are requirement in discrimination claims that the plaintiff show an entire group has been negatively impacted by a workplace policy or general practice.

discriminatory treatment – a requirement in discrimination law that the plaintiff show one person has been harmed by discriminatory practices.

district courts – trial courts in the United States federal court system.

divided custody – form of custody where each parent is awarded sole custody during different parts of the year.

due process – a guarantee that the judicial process will be fair and the trial impartial.

Durham rule – standard for insanity that considers if the crime is a product of mental disease in the defendant. It is also called the product rule.

dynamic factors – risk factors that normally change over the course of time and are more likely to be amenable to treatment or intervention to reduce risk.

emergency commitment – a form of civil commitment where a person can be held for a brief period of time, normally 24 to 48 hours, with few due process protections or the formalities involved in extended commitments.

exhibitionist – a person who suffers from a paraphilia characterized by receiving sexual gratification from exposing one's genitals to others.

extended commitment – a form of civil commitment in which an individual is held for an extended period of time in a psychiatric facility with regular review of their status to assess his or her mental health and dangerousness.

extrafamilial child molester – a person who sexually assaults a child who is not related to the molester.

fact witness – a witness who has direct knowledge of the events at dispute in a case. A fact witness is often referred to as simply a witness or an eyewitness if he or she actually saw the events in dispute.

factual disability – a legal disability that meets the criteria for a disability as stated in the insurance contract such as an illness or injury that prevents a person from carrying out their job or any job.

femicide – the murder of someone who is a woman.

fitness – a term synonymous with competence, commonly used in Canadian law.

fixed battery approach – an approach to conducting neuropsychological assessments in which an examiner administers a standardized set of neuropsychological tests in an identical manner to gain a comprehensive picture of the client.

flexible process approach – an approach to conducting neuropsychological assessments in which an examiner administers unrelated tests that target specific neuropsychological deficits.

forensic assessment instruments – psychological measures intended for use in forensic contexts.

forensic psychology – a branch of psychology characterized as the intersection between the law and clinical psychology by which psychologists attempt to assist the courts in order to resolve legal issues.

forensic relevant instrument – psychological measures that focus on clinical issues, which are more common in the legal system such as psychopathy or future violence but have not been designed specifically to be used in the legal system.

frotteurists – individuals who suffer from a paraphilia characterized by rubbing one's genitals on unsuspecting individuals in public places.

functional abilities – abilities that impact a person's functioning within the legal context and interact with the legal process itself.

grave disability – one of the requirements for civil commitment in some jurisdictions or a component of danger to self in other jurisdictions that is characterized by an inability to care for basic needs such as food, shelter and safety.

hired gun – a negative term used to describe an expert witness that testifies for a particular side in a trial and may be willing to testify to anything that side wishes as a result of being paid for the work.

hostile work harassment – sexual harassment in which sexual demands or behaviors make the work environment unbearable.

idiographic – concerns the study of specific unique events or individuals and normally is used in the context of violence risk assessment.

in absentia – a Latin phrase meaning "in absence" and used to indicate the legal prohibition of an individual being absent from certain legal proceedings.

instrumental violence – violence committed with a purpose or in a planned or organized manner.

intentional torts – a category of torts that indicates an intentional or purposeful act is required for liability such as in cases of assault and battery.

intergenerational transmission of violence – the finding in psychology that victims of violence in one generation (children of violent parents) are more likely to perpetrate violence against the following generation (their own children).

intoxication – a legal defense that claims a person's normal capacity is inhibited by the consumption of alcohol or drugs.

intrafamilial child molester – a person who sexually assaults a child who is related to the molester, or is a member of the molester's family.

irresistible impulse test – a legal requirement for insanity often added to the *M'Naghten* standard that requires a defendant be found insane if his or her behavior was the result of an impulse that the defendant could not control.

joint custody – form of custody where parents share custody of a child or children and both have ongoing responsibility for their care.

joint-degree program – a type of graduate program in which the student earns both a degree in psychology and one in the law simultaneously.

junk science – a termed used in legal rulings to refer to expert testimony based on poor or unsubstantiated findings.

jurisdiction – the power of the court to rule in a matter in a particular geographic region such as a county or state.

juvenile delinquency – behavior that is a violation of criminal law, but is committed by individuals who have not yet become adults.

legal custody – a form of custody that allows the custodian to make legal decisions regarding a child such as for medical treatment.

legal disability – a disability that prevents someone from working because of a license revocation or suspension.

mandatory arrests – a practice requiring law enforcement officials to arrest someone when it is clear that domestic violence has occurred, despite the wishes of the parties involved.

mediation – a legal process by which disputes are resolved through negotiation by a neutral authority figure and not settled in court.

mens rea – a Latin phrase meaning "guilty mind" that is used to indicate intent to commit a crime. The presence of mens rea is a requirement for guilt in many crimes.

meta-analysis – a statistical technique that allows for the quantitative combination of data from numerous studies.

M'Naghten **standard** – insanity standard that applies if the defendant suffers from a defect of reason, from disease of the mind, as not to know the nature and quality of the act or did know he was doing wrong. It is the most frequently used standard in the United States.

negligence – a type of tort in which a person does not act as a reasonable person would under certain circumstances.

nomothetic – refers to the study of universal or general scientific laws that are applicable to groups of people. The term is frequently used in violence risk assessment to contrast with idiographic decisions made about individuals.

objective test – a personality tests in which an individual is asked a question and expected to respond in a structured and direct manner such as on a rating scale or a true/false format.

paraphilia – a broad class of mental illnesses characterized by abnormal sexual thoughts, urges, and behaviors.

paraphilia NOS – a type of paraphilia that does not fall under the specific diagnostic requirements of any other subtype of paraphilia, but is a sexual disorder nonetheless, a paraphilia not otherwise specified.

parens patriae – a Latin phrase meaning "parents of the country" that is the basis of a legal doctrine that encourages the state to act as a parent to anyone in need of protection.

passive avoidance learning – a learning deficit that makes it less likely that psychopaths will inhibit behavior in order to avoid punishment.

pedophile – a person who suffers from a subtype of paraphilia in which the individual reports thoughts, urges, or behaviors indicating sexual attraction toward prepubescent children.

penile plethysmograph – a phallometric method of assessment in sexual offenders that consists of assessing the individual's arousal to sexual stimuli through physiological devices.

persitors – individuals who have committed juvenile crimes and continue their criminal pattern as adults.

physical custody – custody based on the parent the children live with and is primarily responsible for their daily care. Custodial arrangements such as sole custody and joint custody normally refer to the physical custody of the child, not the legal custody.

police power – a legal doctrine that empowers the state to act in a way that is necessary to protect the general welfare of society.

policy evaluator – psychologists who use their training in research methodology to asses the effectiveness of government policies, regulations, and laws.

posttraumatic stress disorder – an anxiety disorder precipitated by a traumatic event that leads to symptoms involving re-experiencing the event, avoidance of event related stimuli, and increased arousal.

prejudicial – causing harm or injury, normally used in the context of the prohibition of evidence that is more prejudicial than probative.

preventative commitment – a form of civil commitment in which an individual does not meet the legal requirements for civil commitment but he or she is expected to deteriorate in the future and will meet the requirement.

primary psychopathy – a subtype of psychopathy in which the individual is free from anxiety and best represents a true psychopath.

probative value – helping to prove a particular point, used in the context of the prohibition of the admission of evidence that is more prejudicial than probative.

procedural justice – a notion that focuses on the process by which decisions are made instead of the outcome of those decisions.

product rule – standard for insanity that considers if the crime is a product of mental disease in the defendant. It is also called the Durham rule.

projective test – a personality test that involves the presentation of ambiguous stimuli.

protective factors – characteristics that reduce the likelihood of someone committing violence or other crimes in the future.

psychopathy – a clinical construct characterized by deficits in interpersonal and emotional functioning that increase the likelihood of the individual behaving in an antisocial manner.

punitive damages – damages awarded in a civil trial in excess of compensatory damages that are intended to punish plaintiffs for their behavior.

quid pro quo harassment – sexual harassment in which an employer or supervisor expects the employee to comply with sexual demands or behaviors in order to maintain their employment.

reactive violence – a form of violence that occurs out of emotion such as anger or fear.

recidivism – repeat criminal behavior normally defined by an additional criminal conviction and subsequent incarceration.

relapse prevention – a form of treatment used with sexual offenders in which the individual is taught to identify situations in which relapse or the commission of a sexual crime is likely to take place in order to avoid those situations.

reliability – a scientific term related to consistency and stability of measurement.

responsivity principle – the idea that any treatment should match the needs of the individual being treated and thereby specifically tailored to him or her in order to increase the likelihood of effectiveness.

Archer, R. P., Buffington-Vollum, J. K., Stredny, R. V., & Handel, R. W. (2006). A survey of psychological test use patterns among forensic psychologists. *Journal of Personality Assessment, 87,* 85–95.

Association of Family and Conciliation Courts. (n.d.). *Model standards of practice for child custody evaluation.* Milwaukee, WI: Author.

Atkins v. Virginia, 536 U.S. 304, 153 L. Ed. 2d 335, 122 S. Ct. 2242 (2002).

Augimeri, L., Koegl, C., Webster, C. D., & Levene, K. (2001). *Early assessment risk list for boys: EARL-20B, Version 2.* Toronto: Earlscourt Child and Family Centre.

Azevedo, D. (1996). Disarming hired guns. *Medical Economics, 73,* 174–183.

Babcock, J. C., Green, C. E., & Robie, C. (2004). Does batterers' treatment work? A meta-analytic review of domestic violence treatment. *Clinical Psychology Review, 23,* 1023–1053.

Babcock, J. C., Miller, S. A., & Siard, C. (2003). Toward a typology of abusive women: Differences between partner-only and generally violent women in the use of violence. *Psychology of Women Quarterly, 27,* 153–161.

Babiak, P., & Hare, R. D. (2006). *Snakes in suits: When psychopaths go to work.* New York: Regan Books/HarperCollins Publishers.

Bagby R. M., Nicholson, R. A., Buis, T., & Bacchiochi, J. R. (2000). Can the MMPI-2 validity scales detect depression feigned by experts? *Assessment, 7,* 55–62.

Banks v. Goodfellow L. R., 5 Q.B. 549 (1870).

Barbaree, H. E. (2005). Psychopathy, treatment behavior, and recidivism: An extended follow-up of Seto and Barbaree. *Journal of Interpersonal Violence, 20,* 1115–1131.

Barbaree, H. E., Seto, M. C., Langton, C. M., & Peacock, E. J. (2001). Evaluating the predicting accuracy of six risk assessment instruments for adult sex offenders. *Criminal Justice and Behavior, 28,* 490–521.

Bardwell, M. C., & Arrigo, B. A. (2002). Competency to stand trial: A law, psychology, and policy assessment. *Journal of Psychiatry and Law, 30,* 147–269.

Barefoot v. Estelle, 462 U.S. 880 (1983).

Barnett, O. W., & Fagan, R. W. (1993). Alcohol use in male spouse abusers and their female partners. *Journal of Family Violence, 8,* 1–25.

Bartel, P., Borum, R., & Forth, A. (2000). *Structured assessment for violence risk in youth (SAVRY).* Tampa, FL: Louis de la Parte Florida Mental Health Institute, University of South Florida.

Barth, J. T., Ruff, R., & Espe-Pfeifer, P. (2005). Mild traumatic brain injury: Definitions. In G. Young, A. W. Kane, & K. Nicholson (Eds.), *Psychological knowledge in court: PTSD, pain, and TBI* (pp. 55–69). New York: Springer.

Baumgartner, J. V., Scalora, M. J., & Huss, M. T. (2002). Assessment of the Wilson Sex Fantasy Questionnaire among child molesters and nonsexual forensic offenders. *Sexual Abuse: Journal of Research and Treatment, 14,* 19–30.

Bauserman, R. (2002). Child adjustment in joint-custody versus sole-custody arrangements: A meta-analytic review. *Journal of Family Psychology, 16,* 91–102.

Becker, J. V., Cunningham-Rather, J., & Kaplan, M. S. (1986). Adolescent sexual offenders: Demographics, criminal and sexual histories, and recommendations for reducing future offenses. *Journal of Interpersonal Violence, 1,* 431–445.

Beckham, J. C., Annis, L. V., & Bein, M. F. (1986). Don't pass go: Predicting who returns from court as remaining incompetent for trial. *Criminal Justice and Behavior, 13,* 99–109.

Beckham, J. C., Annis, L. V., & Gustafson, D. J. (1989). Decision making and examiner bias in forensic expert recommendations for not guilty by reason of insanity. *Law and Human Behavior, 13*, 79–87.

Benjamin, G. A. H., & Gollan, J. K. (2003). *Family evaluation in custody litigation: Reducing risks of ethical infractions and malpractice.* Washington, DC: American Psychological Association.

Benjamin, L. T. (2006). Hugo Münsterberg's attack on the application of scientific psychology. *Journal of Applied Psychology, 91*, 414–425.

Bennett, G. T., & Kish, G. R. (1990). Incompetency to stand trial: Treatment unaffected by demographic variables. *Journal of Forensic Sciences, 35*, 403–412.

Bennett, N. S., Lidz, C. W., Monahan, J., Mulvey, E. P., Hoge, S. K., Roth, L. H., et al. (1993). Inclusion, motivation, and good faith: The morality of coercion in mental hospital admission. *Behavioral Sciences and the Law, 11*, 295–306.

Benson, M. L., Wooldredge, J., Thistlethwaite, A. B., & Fox, G. L. (2004). The correlation between race and domestic violence is confounded with community context. *Social Problems, 51*, 326–342.

Bernet, W. (2002). Child custody evaluations. *Child and Adolescent Psychiatric Clinics of North America, 11*, 781–804.

Berry, D. T. R., & Butcher, J. N. (1998). Detecting of feigning of head injury symptoms on the MMPI-2. In C. R. Reynolds (Ed.), *Critical issues in neuropsychology* (pp. 209–238). New York: Plenum Press.

Bersoff, D. N., Goodman-Delahunty, J., Grisso, J. T., Hans, V. P., Poythress, N. G., & Roesch, R. (1997). Training in law and psychology: Models from the Villanova Conference. *American Psychologist, 52*, 1301–1310.

Bigelow, D. A., Bloom, J. D., Williams, M., & McFarland, B. H. (1999). An administrative model for close monitoring and managing high risk individuals. *Behavioral Sciences and the Law, 17*, 225–237.

Binder, L. M., & Rohling, M. L. (1996). Money matters: Meta-analytic review of the effects of financial incentives on recovery after closed-head injury. *American Journal of Psychiatry, 153*, 7–10.

Bishop, D., & Frazier, C. (2000). Consequences of transfer. In J. Fagan & F. E. Zimring (Eds.), *The changing borders of juvenile justice: Transfer of adolescents to the criminal court* (pp. 227–276). Chicago: University of Chicago Press.

Black, B., & Singer, J. A. (1993). From Frye to Daubert: A new test for scientific evidence. *Shepard's Expert and Science Evidence Quarterly, 1*, 19–39.

Black, D. A., Heyman, R. E., & Slep, A. M. S. (2001). Risk factors for male-to-male partner sexual abuse. *Aggression and Violent Behavior, 6*, 269–280.

Blackburn, R. (1996). What *is* forensic psychology? *Legal and Criminological Psychology, 1*, 3–16.

Blair, R. J. R. (1999). Responsiveness to distress cues in the child with psychopathic tendencies. *Personality and Individual Differences, 27*, 135–145.

Blair, R. J. R., Jones, L., Clark, F., & Smith, M. (1997). The psychopathic individual: A lack of responsiveness to distress cues? *Psychophysiology, 34*, 192–198.

Blanchard, E. B., Hickling, E. J., Taylor, A. E., Loos, W. R., Forneris, C. A., & Jaccard, J. (1996). Who develops from motor vehicle accidents? *Behaviour Research and Therapy, 34*, 1–10.

Blanchard, R., Klassen, P., Dickey, R., Kuban, M. E., & Blak, T. (2001). Sensitivity and specificity of the phallometric test for pedophilia in non admitting sex offenders. *Psychological Assessment, 13*, 118–126.

Blau, T. H. (1998). *The psychologist as expert witness* (2nd ed.). New York: John Wiley & Sons, Inc.

Boccaccini, M. T. (2002). What do we really know about witness preparation. *Behavioral Sciences and the Law, 20,* 161–189.

Boccaccini, M. T., & Brodsky, S. L. (2002). Believability of expert and lay witnesses: Implications for trial consultation. Professional *Psychology: Research and Practice, 33,* 384–388.

Bodholdt, R. H., Richards, H. R., & Gacono, C. B. (2000). Assessing psychopathy in adults: The psychopathy checklist-revised and screening version. In C. B. Gacono (Ed.), *The clinical and forensic assessment of psychopathy: A practitioners guide* (pp. 55–86). Mahwah, NJ: Lawrence Erlbaum Associates.

Boer, D. P., Hart, S. D., Kropp, P. R., & Webster, C. D. (1997). *Manual for the Sexual Violence Risk – 20.* Burnaby, British Columbia: Mental Health, Law, and Policy Institute, Simon Fraser University.

Boothby, J. L., & Clements, C. B. (2000). A national survey of correctional psychologists. *Criminal Justice and Behavior, 27,* 716–732.

Bonnie, R. J., & Grisso, T. (2000). Adjudicative competence and youthful offenders. In T. Grisso, & R. G. Schwartz (Eds.), *Youth on trial: A developmental perspective on juvenile justice* (pp. 73–103). Chicago: University of Chicago Press.

Bonsack, C., & Borgeat, F. (2005). Perceived coercion and need for hospitalization related to psychiatric admission. *International Journal of Law and Psychiatry, 28,* 342–347.

Borum, R. (1996). Improving the clinical practice of violence risk assessment: Technology, guidelines, and training. *American Psychologist, 51,* 945–956.

Borum, R. (2000). Assessing violence risk among youth. *Journal of Clinical Psychology, 56,* 1263–1288.

Borum, R. (2003a). Managing at-risk juvenile offenders in the community. *Journal of Contemporary Criminal Justice, 19,* 114–137.

Borum, R. (2003b). Not guilty by reason of insanity. In T. Grisso (Ed.), *Evaluating competencies: Forensic assessments and instruments* (2nd ed., pp. 193–228). New York: Kluwer/Plenum.

Borum, R., & Fulero, S. M. (1999). Empirical research on the insanity defense and attempted reforms: Evidence toward informed policy. *Law and Human Behavior, 23,* 117–135.

Borum, R., & Grisso, T. (1995). Psychological test use in criminal forensic evaluations. *Professional Psychology: Research and Practice, 26,* 465–473.

Borum, R., & Grisso, T. (1996). Establishing standards for criminal forensic reports: An empirical analysis. *Bulletin of the American Academy of Psychiatry & the Law, 24,* 297–317.

Borum, R., & Otto, R. (2000). Advances in forensic assessment and treatment. *Law and Human Behavior, 24,* 1–7.

Bottoms v. Bottoms, 249 Va. 410, 457 S.E. 2d 102 (1995).

Bottoms, B., Costanzo, M., Greene, E., Redlich, A., Woolard, J., & Zapf, P. (2004). Careers in Psychology and the Law: A guide for prospective students. Available online at http://ap-ls.org/students/careers%20in%20psychology.pdf

Bow, J. N., & Quinnell, F. A. (2001). Psychologists' current practices and procedures in child custody evaluations: Five years after American Psychological Association guidelines. *Professional Psychology: Research, and Practice, 32,* 261–268.

Bow, J. N., Quinnell, F. A., Zarnoff, M., & Assemany, A. (2002). Assessment of sexual abuse allegations in child custody cases. *Professional Psychology: Research and Practice, 33*, 566–575.

Bowie v. Arder, 476 N. W. 2d 649 (1991).

Boyle, D. J., & Vivian, D. (1996). Generalized versus spouse-specific anger/hostility and men's violence against intimates. *Violence and Victims, 11*, 293–317.

Bradford, J. M. W. (1985). Organic treatments for the male sexual offender. *Behavioral Sciences and the Law, 3*, 355–375.

Bradley, A. (2003). Child custody evaluations. In W. T. O'Donohue & E. R. Levensky (Eds.), *Handbook of forensic psychology: Resource for mental health and legal professionals* (pp. 234–243). New York: Elsevier.

Braff, J., Arvanites, T., & Steadman, H. J. (1983). Detention patters of successful and unsuccessful insanity defendants. *Criminology, 21*, 439–448.

Brakel, S. J., Parry, J., & Weiner, B. (1985). *The mentally disabled and the law* (3rd ed.). Chicago: American Bar Foundation.

Brewer, N., & Williams, K. (2005). *Psychology and law: An empirical perspective.* New York: Guilford.

Bricklin, B. (1989). *Perception of relationships test manual.* Furlong, PA: Village Publishing.

Bricklin, B. (1990a). *Bricklin perceptual scales manual.* Furlong, PA: Village Publishing.

Bricklin, B. (1990b). *Parent awareness skills survey manual.* Furlong, PA: Village Publishing.

Bricklin, B., & Elliot, G. (1991). *Parent perception of child profile manual.* Furlong, PA: Village Publishing.

Brigham, J. C. (1999). What is forensic psychology, anyway? *Law and Human Behavior, 23*, 273–298.

Brinkley, C. A., Bernstein, A., & Newman, J. P. (1999). Coherence in the narratives of psychopathic and nonpsychopathic criminal offenders. *Personality and Individual Differences, 27*, 519–530.

Brodin, M. S. (2005). Behavioral science evidence in the age of Daubert: Reflections of a skeptic. *University of Cincinnati Law Review, 73*, 867–943.

Brodsky, S. L. (1991). *Testifying in court: Guidelines and maxims for the expert witness.* Washington, DC: American Psychological Association.

Brodsky, S. L., & Bennett, A. L. (2005). Psychological assessments of confessions and suggestibility in mentally retarded suspects. *Journal of Psychiatry and Law, 33*, 359–366.

Brodsky, S. L., Caputo, A. A., & Domino, M. L. (2002). The mental health professionals in court. In B. Van Dorsten (Ed.), *Forensic psychology: From classroom to courtroom* (pp. 17–33). New York: Kluwer Academic/Plenum.

Brodzinsky, D. M. (1993). On the use and misuse of psychological testing in child custody evaluations. *Professional Psychology: Research and Practice, 24*, 213–219.

Brown, D. R. (1992). A didactic group program for persons found unfit to stand trial. *Hospital & Community Psychiatry, 43*, 732–733.

Brown, S. L., & Forth, A. E. (1997). Psychopathy and sexual assault: Static risk factors, emotional precursors, and rapist subtypes. *Journal of Consulting and Clinical Psychology, 65*, 848–857.

Bullock, J. L. (2003). Involuntary treatment of defendants found incompetent to stand trial. *Journal of Forensic Psychology Practice, 2*, 1–33.

DeMatteo, D., & Edens, J. F. (2006). The role and relevance of the Psychopathy Checklist-Revised in court: A case law survey of U.S. courts (1991–2004). *Psychology, Public Policy, and Law, 12,* 214–241.

DeMatteo, D., & Marczyk, G. (2005). Risk factors, protective factors, and the prevention of antisocial behavior among juveniles. In K. Heilbrun, N. E. S. Goldstein, & R. E. Redding, *Juvenile delinquency: Prevention, assessment, and intervention* (pp. 19–44). New York: Oxford University Press.

Department of Health and Human Services. (2001). *Youth violence: A report of the Surgeon General.* Rockville, MD: Author.

Dersh, J., Polatin, P., & Gatchel, R. (2002). Chronic pain and psychopathology: Research findings and theoretical considerations. *Psychosomatic Medicine, 64,* 773–786.

Devenport, J. L., & Cutler, B. L. (2004). Impact of defense-only and opposing eyewitness experts on juror judgments. *Law and Human Behavior, 28,* 569–576.

DeVoe, J. F., Ruddy, S. A., Miller, A. K., Planty, M. Snyder, T. D., Peter, K., et al. (2002). *Indicators of school crime and safety: 2002.* (NCES 2003-0009/NCJ196753). Washington, DC: U.S. Department of Education and Justice, American Institutes of Research.

de Vogel, V., De Ruiter, C., & van Beek, D., & Mead, G. (2004). Predictive validity of the SVR-20 and Static-99 in a Dutch sample of treated sex offenders. *Law and Human Behavior, 28,* 235–251.

Dirks-Linhorst, P. A., & Linhorst, D. M. (2006). A description of the design and costs of an insanity acquittee conditional release, monitoring, and revocation system. *International Journal of Forensic Mental Health, 5,* 55–65.

Dobash R. E., & Dobash, R. P. (1979). *Violence against wives: A case against the patriarchy.* New York: The Free Press.

Doren, D. M. (2002). *Evaluating sex offenders: A manual for civil commitments and beyond.* Thousand Oaks, CA: Sage.

Doren, D. M. (2004). Toward a multidimensional model for sexual recidivism risk. *Journal of Interpersonal Violence, 19,* 835–856.

Dorfman, L., & Shiraldi, V. (2001, April). *Off balance: Youth, race, and crime in the news.* Washington, DC: Building Blocks for Youth Initiative.

Douglas, K. S., & Dutton, D. G. (2001). Assessing the link between stalking and domestic violence. *Aggression and Violent Behavior, 6,* 519–546.

Douglas, K. S., Huss, M. T., Murdoch, L. L., Washington, D. O., & Koch, W. J. (1999). Posttraumatic stress disorder stemming from motor vehicle accidents: Legal issues in Canada and the United States. In E. J. Hickling & E. B. Blanchard (Eds.), *The international handbook of road traffic accidents & psychological trauma: Current understanding, treatment and law* (pp. 271–289). New York: Elsevier Science.

Douglas, K. S., & Koch, W. J. (2001a). Civil commitment and civil competence: Psychological issues. In R. A. Schuller, & J. R. P Ogloff, *Introduction to psychology and law: Canadian perspectives* (pp. 353–374). Toronto: University of Toronto Press.

Douglas, K. S., & Koch, W. J. (2001b). Psychological injuries and tort litigation: Sexual victimization and motor vehicle accidents. In R. A. Schuller & J. R. P. Ogloff (Eds.), *Introduction to psychology and law: Canadian perspectives* (pp. 405–425). Toronto: University of Toronto Press.

Douglas, K. S., & Ogloff, J. R. P. (2003). Multiple facets of risk for violence: The impact of judgmental specificity on structured decisions about violence risk. *International Journal of Forensic Mental Health, 2,* 19–34.

Douglas, K. S., Ogloff, J. R. P., Nicholls, T. L., & Grant, I. (1999). Assessing risk for violence among psychiatric patients: The HCR-20 violence risk assessment scheme and the Psychopathy Checklist: Screening Version. *Journal of Consulting and Clinical Psychology, 67*, 917–930.

Douglas, K. S., & Skeem, J. L. (2005). Violence risk assessment: Getting specific about being dynamic. *Psychology, Public Policy, and Law, 11*, 347–383

Douglas, K. S., & Webster, C. D. (1999). The HCR-20 violence risk assessment scheme: Concurrent validity in a sample of incarcerated offenders. *Criminal Justice and Behavior, 26*, 3–19.

Douglas, K. S., Yeomans, M., & Boer, D. P. (2005). Comparative validity analysis of multiple measures of violence risk in a sample of criminal offenders. *Criminal Justice and Behavior, 32*, 479–510.

Dowden, C., & Andrews, D. A. (2000). Effective correctional treatment and violent reoffending: A meta-analysis. *Canadian Journal of Criminology, 42*, 449–467.

Dowden, C., Antonowicz, D., & Andrews, D. A. (2003). The effectiveness of relapse prevention with offenders: A meta-analysis. *International Journal of Offender Therapy and Comparative Criminology, 47*, 516–528.

Doyle, J. M. (2005). *True witness: Cops, courts, science, and the battle against misidentification.* New York: Palgrave.

Doyle, M., Dolan, M., & McGovern, J. (2002). The validity of North American risk assessment tools in predicting in-patient violent behaviour in England. *Legal and Criminological Psychology, 7*, 141–154.

Drogin, E. Y., & Barrett, C. L. (2007). Off the witness stand: The forensic psychologist as consultant. In A. M. Goldstein (Ed.), *Forensic psychology: Emerging topics and expanding roles* (pp. 465 – 488). Hoboken, NJ: John Wiley & Sons.

Drope v. Missouri, 420 U.S. 162, 95 S.Ct. 896 (1975).

D'Silva, K., Duggan, C., & McCarthy, L. (2004). Does treatment really make psychopaths worse? A review of the evidence. *Journal of Personality Disorders, 18*, 163–177.

Durham v. United States, 214 F.2d 862 (1954).

Dush, D. M., Simons, L. E., Platt, M., Nation, P. C., & Ayres, S. Y. (1994). Psychological profiles distinguishing litigating and nonlitigating pain patients: Subtle, and not so subtle. *Journal of Personality Assessment, 62*, 299–313.

Dusky v. United States, 362 U.S. 402, 80 S.Ct. 788 (1960).

Dutton, D. G. (2002). Personality dynamics of intimate abusiveness. *Journal of Psychiatric Practice, 8*, 216–228.

Dutton, D. G., & Kropp, P. R. (2000). A review of domestic violence risk instruments. *Trauma, Violence, & Abuse, 1*, 171–181.

Dutton, D. G., Starzomski, A., & Ryan, L. (1996). Antecedents of abusive personality and abusive behavior in wife assaulters. *Journal of Family Violence, 11*, 113–132.

Dvoskin, J. A., & Spiers, E. M. (2004). On the role of correctional officers in prison mental health. *Psychiatric Quarterly, 75*, 41–59.

Edens, J. F. (2001). Misuses of the Hare Psychopathy Checklist-Revised in court. *Journal of Interpersonal Violence, 16*, 1082–1093.

Edens, J. F. (2006). Unresolved controversies concerning psychopathy: Implications for clinical and forensic decision making. *Professional Psychology: Research and Practice, 37*, 59–65.

Edens, J. F., Buffington-Vollum, J. K., & Keilen, A., Roskamp, P., & Anthony, C. D. (2005). Predictions of future dangerousness in capital murder trials: Is it time to "disinvent the wheel?" *Law and Human Behavior, 29*, 55–86.

Grisso, T. (2004). Reply to "a critical review of published competency-to-confess measures." *Law and Human Behavior, 28,* 719–724.

Grisso, T., & Appelbaum, P. S. (1995). The MacArthur Treatment Competence Study: II. Measures of abilities related to competence to consent to treatment. *Law and Human Behavior, 19,* 127–148.

Grisso, T., & Appelbaum, P. S. (1998). *MacArthur competence assessment tool for treatment (MacCAT-T).* Sarasota, FL: Professional Resource Press.

Grisso, T., Cocozza, J. J., Steadman, H. J., Greer, A., & Fisher, W. H. (1996). A national survey of hospital and community-based approaches to pretrial mental health evaluations. *Psychiatric Services, 47,* 642–644.

Grisso, T., Davis, J., Vesselinov, R., Appelbaum, P. S., & Monahan, J. (2000). Violent thoughts and violent behavior following hospitalization for mental disorder. *Journal of Consulting and Clinical Psychology, 68,* 388–398.

Grisso, T., Steinberg, L., Woolard, J., Cauffman, E., Scott, E., Graham, S., et al. (2003). Juveniles competence to stand trial: A comparison of adolescents' and adults' capacities as trial defendants. *Law and Human Behavior, 27,* 333–363.

Groscup, J. L., Penrod, S. D., Studebaker, C. A., Huss, M. T., & O'Neil, K. M. (2002). The effects of Daubert on the admissibility of expert testimony in state and federal criminal cases. *Psychology, Public Policy, and Law, 8,* 339–372.

Grubin, D. (1999). Actuarial and clinical assessment of risk in sex offenders. *Journal of Interpersonal Violence, 14,* 331–343.

Guerrero, J., Thurman, D. J., & Sniezek, J. E. (2000). Emergency department visits associated with traumatic brain injury: United States, 1995–1996. *Brain Injury, 14,* 181–186.

Gunnoe, M. L., & Braver, S. L. (2001). The effects of joint legal custody on mothers, fathers, and children controlling for factors that predispose a sole maternal versus joint legal award. *Law and Human Behavior, 25,* 25–43.

Gutheil, T. G. (1999). A confusion of tongues: Competence, insanity, psychiatry, and the law. *Psychiatric Services, 50,* 767–773.

Gutheil, T. G., & Simon, R. I. (1999). Attorneys' pressure on the expert witness: Early warning signs of endangered honesty, objectivity, and fair competition. *Journal of the American Academy of Psychiatry and the Law, 27,* 546–553.

Gutheil, T. G., & Simon, R. I. (2004). Avoiding bias in expert testimony. *Psychiatric Annals, 34,* 260–270.

Gutheil, T. G., & Sutherland, P. K. (1999). Forensic assessment, witness credibility and the search for truth through expert testimony in the courtroom. *Journal of Psychiatry & Law, 27,* 289–312.

Guy, L. S., & Douglas, K. S. (2006). Examining the utility of the PCL: SV as a screening measure using competing factor models of psychopathy. *Psychological Assessment, 18,* 225–230.

Guy, L. S., Edens, J. F., Anthony, C., & Douglas, K. S. (2005). Does psychopathy predict institutional misconduct among adults? A meta-analytic investigation. *Journal of Consulting and Clinical Psychology, 73,* 1056–1064.

Guyer, C. G. (2000). Spouse abuse. In F. W. Kaslow (Ed.), *Handbook of couple and family forensics: A sourcebook for mental health and legal professionals* (pp. 206–234). Hoboken, NJ: John Wiley & Sons.

Haas, L. J. (1993). Competence and quality in the performance of forensic psychologists. *Ethics & Behavior, 3,* 251–266.

Hagen, M. (1997). *Whores of the court: The fraud of psychiatric testimony and the rape of American justice*. New York: Regan Books.

Hall, A. S., Pulver, C. A., & Cooley, M. J. (1996). Psychology of best interest standard: Fifty state statutes and their theoretical antecedents. *The American Journal of Family Therapy, 24,* 171–180.

Hall, G. C. N. (1995). Sexual offender recidivism revisited: A meta-analysis of recent treatment studies. *Journal of Clinical and Consulting Psychology, 63,* 802–809.

Hall, G. C. N., Proctor, W. C., & Nelson, G. M. (1988). Validity of physiological measures of pedophilic sexual arousal in a sexual offender population. *Journal of Consulting and Clinical Psychology, 56,* 118–122.

Haller, L. H. (2000). Forensic aspects of juvenile violence. *Child and Adolescent Psychiatric Clinics of North America, 9,* 859–881.

Hamparian, D. M., Schuster, R., Dinitz, S., & Conrad, J. P. (1978). *The violent few: A study of dangerous juvenile offenders*. Lexington, MA: Heath.

Haney, C. (1980). Psychology and legal change: On the limits of a factual jurisprudence. *Law and Human Behavior, 4,* 147–199.

Hanscom, D., & Jex, R. (2001). Sleep disorder, depression, and musculoskeletal pain. *Spineline*, Sept/Oct, 20–31.

Hanson, R. K. (2002). Recidivism and age: Follow-up data from 4,673 sexual offenders. *Journal of Interpersonal Violence, 17,* 1046–1062.

Hanson, R. K., & Bussière, M. T. (1998). Predicting relapse: A meta-analysis of sexual offender recidivism studies. *Journal of Consulting and Clinical Psychology, 66,* 348–362.

Hanson, R. K., Cadsky, O., Harris, A., & Lalonde, C. (1997). Correlates of battering among 997 men: Family history, adjustment, and attitudinal differences. *Violence and Victims, 12,* 191–208.

Hanson, R. K., Gordon, A., Harris, A. J., Marques, J. K., Murphy, W., & Quinsey, V. L., et al. (2002). First report of the collaborative data project on the effectiveness of psychological treatment for sex offenders. *Sexual Abuse: A Journal of Research and Treatment, 14,* 169–194.

Hanson, R. K., & Harris, A. J. R. (2000). Where should we intervene? Dynamic predictors of sexual offense recidivism. *Criminal Justice and Behavior, 27,* 6–35.

Hanson, R. K., Morton, K. E., & Harris, A. J. R. (2003). Sexual offender recidivism risk: What we know and what we need to know. *Annals of the New York Academy of Sciences, 989,* 154–166.

Hanson, R. K., & Morton-Bourgon, K. E. (2005). The characteristics of persistent sexual offenders: A meta-analysis of recidivism studies. *Journal of Consulting and Clinical Psychology, 73,* 1154–1163.

Hare, R. D. (1991). *The Hare Psychopathy Checklist-Revised*. Toronto: Multi-Health Systems.

Hare, R. D. (1996). Psychopathy: A clinical construct whose time has come. *Criminal Justice and Behavior, 23,* 25–54.

Hare, R. D. (1999). *Without conscience: The disturbing world of the psychopaths among us*. New York: Guilford.

Hare, R. D. (2001). Psychopaths and their nature: Some implications for understanding human predator violence. In A. Raine & J. Sanmartin (Eds.), *Violence and psychopathy* (pp. 5–34). New York: Kluwer Academic/Plenum Publishers.

Hare, R. D. (2003). *The Hare Psychopathy Checklist-Revised* (2nd ed.). Toronto: Multi-Health Systems.

Hare, R. D., Clark, D., Grann, M., & Thorton, D. (2000). Psychopathy and the predictive validity of the PCL-R: An international perspective. *Behavioral Sciences & the Law, 18*, 623–645.

Hare, R. D., & Hart, S. F. (1996). *Psychopathy and the PCL-R: Clinical and forensic application.* Toronto: Multi-Health Systems.

Hare, R. D., & Neumann, C. S. (2006). The PCL-R assessment of psychopathy: Development, structural properties, and new directions. In C. J. Patrick (Ed.), *Handbook of psychopathy* (pp. 58–88). New York: Guilford Press.

Hare, R. D., McPherson, L. M., & Forth, A. E. (1988). Male psychopaths and their criminal career. *Journal of Consulting and Clinical Psychology, 56*, 710–714.

Hare, R. D., Williamson, S. E., & Harpur, T. J. (1988). Psychopathy and language. In T. E. Moffitt, & S. A Mednick, *Biological contributions to crime causation* (pp. 66–92). Dordrecht, Netherlands: Martinus Nijhoff Publishing.

Harris, A., Phenix, A., Hanson, R. K., & Thorton, D. (2003). *Static-99 coding rules: Revised–2003.* Ottawa, Canada: Solicitor General of Canada.

Harris, G. T., & Rice, M. E. (1997). Mentally disordered offenders: What research says about effective service. In C. D. Webster & M. A. Jackson (Ed.), *Impulsivity: Theory, assessment, and treatment* (pp. 361–393). New York, Guilford Press.

Harris, G. T., & Rice, M. E. (2006). Treatment of psychopathy: A review of empirical findings. In C. J. Patrick (Ed.), *Handbook of psychopathy* (pp. 555–572). New York: Guilford Press.

Harris, G. T., Rice, M. E., & Cormier, C. A. (1991). Psychopathy and violent recidivism. *Law and Human Behavior, 15*, 625–637.

Harris, G. T., Rice, M. E., & Cormier, C. A. (2002). Prospective replication of the Violence Risk Appraisal Guide in predicting violent recidivism among forensic patients. *Law and Human Behavior, 26*, 377–394.

Harris, G. T., Rice, M. E., & Quinsey, V. L. (1993). Violent recidivism of mentally disordered offenders: The development of a statistical prediction instrument. *Criminal Justice and Behavior, 20*, 315–335.

Harris, G. T., Rice, M. E., & Quinsey, V. L. (1998). Appraisal and management of risk in sexual aggressors: Implications for criminal justice policy. *Psychology, Public Policy, and Law, 4*, 73–115.

Hart, S. F. (1998). The role of psychopathy in assessing risk for violence: Conceptual and methodological issues. *Legal and Criminological Psychology, 3*, 121–137.

Hart, S. D. (2005). *Advances in spousal violence risk assessment.* Retrieved on June 14, 2006 from http://dcj.state.co.us/odvsom/Domestic_Violence/DV_Pdfs/Hart-Presentation052504.pdf

Hart, S. D., & Hare, R. D. (1992). Predicting fitness to stand trial: The relative power of demographic, criminal, and clinical variables. *Forensic Reports, 5*, 53–65.

Hart, S. F., & Dempster, R. J. (1997). Impulsivity and psychopathy. In C. D. Webster & M. A. Jackson (Eds.), *Impulsivity: Theory, assessment, and treatment* (pp. 212–232). New York: Guilford Press.

Hart, S. F., Forth, A. E., & Hare, R. D. (1990). Performance of criminal psychopaths on selected neuropsychological tests. *Journal of Abnormal Psychology, 99*, 374–379.

Hart, S. F., Michie, C., & Cooke, D. J. (2007). Precision of actuarial risk assessment instruments: Evaluating the "margins of error" of group v, individual predictions of violence. *British Journal of Psychiatry, 190*, 60–65.

Harvey, A. G., & Bryant, R. A. (2000). Memory for acute stress disorder symptoms: A two-year prospective study. *Journal of Nervous and Mental Disease, 1888,* 602–607.

Heckert, D. A., & Gondolf, E. W. (2000). Assessing assault self-reports by batterer program participants and their partners. *Journal of Family Violence, 15,* 181–197.

Heckert, D. A., & Gondolf, E. W. (2004). Battered women's perceptions of risk versus risk factors and instruments in predicting repeat reassault. *Journal of Interpersonal Violence, 19,* 778–800.

Heilbrun, K. (1987). The assessment of competency for execution: An overview. *Behavioral Sciences and the Law, 5,* 383–396.

Heilbrun, K. (1997). Prediction versus management models relevant to risk assessment: The importance of legal decision-making context. *Law and Human Behavior, 21,* 347–359.

Heilbrun, K. (2003). Developing principles of forensic mental health assessment. In K. Heilbrun (Ed.), *Principles of forensic mental health assessment* (pp. 3–18). New York: Kluwer Academic/Plenum.

Heilbrun, K., & Collins, S. (1995). Evaluation of trial competency and mental state at the time of offense report characteristics. *Professional Psychology: Research and Practice, 26,* 61–67.

Heilbrun, K., & Griffin, P. (1999). Forensic assessment: A review of programs and research. In R. Roesch, S. Hart, & J. R. P. Ogloff (Eds.), *Psychology and the law: State of the discipline* (pp. 242–278). Dordrecht, The Netherlands: Kluwer Academic/Plenum Publishers.

Heilbrun, K., Hart, S., Hare, R. D., Gustafson, D., Nunez, C., & White, A. (1998). Inpatient and post discharge aggression in mentally disordered offenders. *Journal of Interpersonal Violence, 13,* 514–526.

Heilbrun, K., Lee, R. J., & Cottle, C. C. (2005). Risk factors and intervention outcomes: Meta-analyses of juvenile offending. In K. Heilbrun, N. E. S. Goldstein, & R. E. Redding (Eds.), *Juvenile delinquency: Prevention, assessment, and intervention* (pp. 3–18). New York: Oxford University Press.

Heilbrun, K., O'Neil, M. L., Strohman, L. K., Bowman, Q., & Philipson, J. (2000). Expert approaches to communicating violence risk. *Law and Human Behavior, 24,* 137–148.

Heilbrun, K., Rogers, R., & Otto, R. (2002). Forensic assessment: Current status and future directions. In J. R. P. Ogloff (Ed.), *Taking psychology and law into the twenty-first century* (pp. 119–146). New York: Kluwer Academic/Plenum Publishers.

Heinze, M. C., & Grisso, T. (1996). Review of instruments assessing parenting competencies used in child custody evaluations. *Behavioral Sciences and the Law, 14,* 293–313.

Hemphill, J., & Hare, R. D. (2004). Some misconceptions about the Hare PCL-R and risk assessment: A reply to Gendreau, Goggin, and Smith. *Criminal Justice and Behavior, 31,* 203–243.

Hemphill, J., Hare, R. D., & Wong, S. (1998). Psychopathy and recidivism: A review. *Legal and Criminological Psychology, 3,* 139–170.

Hemphill, J. F., & Hart, S. F. (2003). Forensic and clinical issues in the assessment of psychopathy. In A. M. Goldstein (Ed.), *Handbook of psychology: Vol. 11. Forensic psychology* (pp. 87–107). Hoboken, NJ: John Wiley & Sons.

Henggeler, S. W., Rowland, M. D., Randall, J., Ward, D. M., Pickrel, S, G., Cunningham, et al. (1999). Home-based multisystemic therapy as an alternative to the

Julian, T. W., & McKenry, P. C. (1993). Mediators of male violence toward female intimates. *Journal of Family Violence, 8,* 39–56.

Kansas v. Crane, 122 S. Ct. 867 (2002).

Kansas v. Hendricks, 117 S. Ct. 2072 (1997).

Kantor, G. K., & Straus, M. A. (1990). Response of victims to the police and police to the assaults on wives. In M. A. Straus & R. J. Gelles (Eds.), *Physical violence in American families* (pp. 473–487). New Brunswick, NJ: Transaction Publishers.

Kantor, G. K., Jasinski, J. L., & Aldarondo, E. (1994). Sociocultural status and incidence of marital violence in Hispanic families. *Violence and Victims, 9,* 207–222.

Keefe, B., & Pinals, D. A. (2004). Durable power of attorney for psychiatric care. *Journal of the American Academy of Psychiatry and the Law, 32,* 202–204.

Keilin, W. G., & Bloom, L. J. (1986). Child custody evaluation practices: A survey of experienced professionals. *Professional Psychology: Research and Practice, 17,* 338–346.

Kelly, J. B. (2000). Children's adjustment in conflicted marriage and divorce: A decade of review of research. *Journal of the American Academy of Child and Adolescent Psychiatry, 39,* 93–973.

Kemp, A., Green, B. L., Hovanitz, C., & Rawlings, E. I. (1995). Incidence and correlates of posttraumatic stress disorder in battered women: Shelter and community samples. *Journal of Interpersonal Violence, 10,* 43–55.

Kendall, W. D. B., & Cheung, M. (2004). Sexually violent predators and civil commitment laws. *Journal of Child Sexual Abuse, 13,* 41–57.

Kent v. United States, 383 U.S. 541 (1966).

Kiehl, K. A., Smith, A. M., Mendrek, A., Forster, B. B., Hare, R. D., & Liddle, P. F. (2004). Temporal lobe abnormalities in semantic processing by criminal psychopaths as revealed by functional magnetic resonance imaging. *Psychiatry Research: Neuroimaging, 130,* 27–42.

Kiesler, C. A., & Simpkins, C. G. (1993). *The unnoticed majority in psychiatric inpatient care.* New York: Plenum Press.

Klassen, D., & O'Connor, W. A. (1988a). A prospective study of predictors of *violence* in adult male mental health admissions. *Law and Human Behavior, 12,* 143–158.

Klassen, D., & O'Connor, W. A. (1988b). Predicting violence in schizophrenic and non-schizophrenic patients: A prospective study. *Journal of Community Psychology, 16,* 217–227.

Klassen, D., & O'Connor, W. A. (1990). Assessing the risk of violence in released mental patients: A cross validation study. *Psychological Assessment: A Journal of Consulting and Clinical Psychology, 1,* 75–81.

Knapp, S., & VandeCreek, L. (2001). Ethical issues in personality assessment in forensic psychology. *Journal of Personality Assessment, 77,* 242–254.

Knapp, S., & VandeCreek, L. (2006). Forensic psychology. In S. Knapp and L. VandeCreek, Practical ethics for psychologists: A positive approach (pp. 161–173). Washington, DC: American Psychological Association.

Knight, R. A., & Guay, J. (2006). The role of psychopathy in sexual coercion against women. In C. J. Patrick (Ed.), *Handbook of psychopathy* (pp. 512–532). New York: Guilford Press.

Koch, W. J., & Douglas, K. S. (2001). Psychology's intersection with family law. In R. A. Schuller, & J. R. P. Ogloff (Eds.), *Introduction to psychology and law: Canadian perspectives* (pp. 375–406). Toronto: University of Toronto Press.

Koch, W. J., O'Neil, M., & Douglas, K. S. (2005). Empirical limits for the forensic assessment of PTSD litigants. *Law and Human Behavior, 29,* 121–149.

Kosson, D. S. (1996). Psychopathy and dual-task performance under focusing conditions. *Journal of Abnormal Psychology, 105,* 391–400.

Kosson, D. S., & Newman, J. P. (1986). Psychopathy and the allocation of attentional capacity in a divided-attention situation. *Journal of Abnormal Psychology, 95,* 257–263.

Kosson, D. S., Smith, S. S., & Newman, J. P. (1990). Evaluating the construct validity of psychopathy in Black and White male inmates: Three preliminary studies. *Journal of Abnormal Psychology, 99,* 250–259.

Kozol, H., Boucher, R., & Garofalo, R. (1972). The diagnosis and treatment of dangerousness. *Crime and Delinquency, 18,* 371–392.

Krauss, D. A., & Sales, B. D. (2000). Legal standards, expertise, and experts in the resolution of contested child custody cases. *Psychology, Public Policy, and Law, 6,* 843–879.

Kravitz, H. H., & Kelly, J. (1999). An outpatient psychiatry program for offenders with mental disorders found not guilty by reason of insanity. *Psychiatric Services, 50,* 1597–1605.

Kress, K. (2000). An argument for assisted outpatient treatment for persons with serious mental illness illustrated with reference to a proposed statute for Iowa. *Iowa Law Review, 85,* 1269–1386.

Krisberg, B., & Wolf, A. M. (2005). Juvenile offending. In K. Heilbrun, N. E. S. Goldstein, & R. E. Redding, *Juvenile delinquency: Prevention, assessment, and intervention* (pp. 67–84). New York: Oxford University Press.

Kropp, P. R., & Hart, S. D. (2000). The spousal assault risk assessment (SARA) guide: Reliability and validity in adult male offenders. *Law and Human Behavior, 24,* 101–118.

Kropp, P. R., Hart, S. D., Webster, C. D., & Eaves, D. (1998). *Spousal assault risk assessment: User's guide.* Toronto: Multi-Health System Inc. and British Columbia Institute Against Family Violence.

Kumho Tire Co., Ltd. v. Carmichael, 119 S. Ct. 1167 (1999).

Kurtz, A. (2002). What works for delinquency? The effectiveness of interventions for teenage offending behaviour, *The Journal of Forensic Psychiatry, 13,* 671–692.

La Fond, J. Q. (2003). Outpatient commitment's next frontier: Sexual predators. *Psychology, Public Policy, and Law, 9,* 159–182.

Ladds, B., & Convit, A. (1994). Involuntary medication of patients who are incompetent to stand trial: A review of empirical studies. *Bulletin of the American Academy of Psychiatry & the Law, 22,* 519–532.

Lake v. Cameron, 364 F.2d. 657 (1966).

Lally, S. J. (2003). What tests are acceptable for use in forensic evaluations? A survey of experts. *Professional Psychology: Research and Practice, 34,* 491–498.

Lalumière, M. L., Harris, G. T., Quinsey, V. L., & Rice, M. E. (2005). *The causes of rape: Understanding individual differences in male propensity for sexual aggression.* Washington DC, American Psychological Association.

Lalumière, M., & Quinsey, V. L. (1994). The discriminability of rapists from non rapists using phallometric measures: A meta-analysis. *Criminal Justice and Behavior, 21,* 150–175.

Lamb, H. R., & Grant, R. W. (1982). The mentally ill in an urban county jail. *Archives of General Psychiatry, 39,* 17–22.

Landenberger, N. A., & Lipsey, M. W. (2005). The positive effects of cognitive-behavioral programs for offenders: A meta-analysis of factors associated with effective treatment. *Journal of Experimental Criminology, 1*, 451–476.

Langelier, P., & Nurcombe, B. (1985). Residual parental rights: Legal trends and controversies. *Journal of the American Academy of Child Psychiatry, 24*, 793–796.

Langevin, R., Curnoe, S., & Bain, J. (2000). A study of clerics who commit sexual offenses: Are they different from other sex offenders? *Child Abuse & Neglect, 24*, 535–545.

Langton, C. M., & Marshall, W. L. (2001). Cognition in rapists: Theoretical patterns by typological breakdown. *Aggression and Violent Behavior, 6*, 499–518.

Langhinrichsen-Rohling, J. (2005). Top 10 greatest "hits": Important findings and future directions for intimate partner violence research. *Journal of Interpersonal Violence, 20*, 108–118.

Langhinrichsen-Rohling, J., Huss, M. T., & Ramsey, S. (2000). The clinical utility of batterer typologies. *Journal of Family Violence, 15*, 37–54.

Langhinrichsen-Rohling, J., Huss, M. T., & Rohling, M. L. (2006). Aggressive behavior. In M. Hersen (Ed.), *Clinician's handbook of adult behavioral assessment* (pp. 371–400). San Diego: Elsevier Academic Press.

Langhinrichsen-Rohling, J., Palarea, R. E., Cohen, J., & Rohling, M. L. (2000). Breaking up is hard to do: Unwanted pursuit behaviors following the dissolution of a romantic relationship. *Violence and Victims, 15*, 73–90.

Leavitt, N., & Maykuth, P. L. (1989). Conformance to attorney performance standards: Advocacy behavior in a maximum security prison hospital. *Law and Human Behavior, 13*, 217–230.

Lees-Haley, P. R. (1997). MMPI-2 base rates for 492 personal injury plaintiffs: Implications and challenges for forensic assessment. *Journal of Clinical Psychology, 53*, 745–755.

Lees-Haley, P. R. (1992). Neuropsychological complaint base rates of personal injury claimants. *Forensic Reports, 5*, 385–391.

Lees-Haley, P. R., Smith, H. R., Williams, C. W., & Dunn, J. T. (1996). Forensic neuropsychological test usage: An empirical survey. *Archives of Clinical Neuropsychology, 11*, 45–51.

Leisring, P. A., Dowd, L., & Rosenbaum, A. (2003). Treatment of partner aggressive women. *Journal of Aggression, Maltreatment & Trauma, 7*, 257–277.

Leonard, K. E., & Blane, H. T. (1992). Alcohol and marital aggression in a national sample of young men. *Journal of Interpersonal Violence, 7*, 19–30.

Leonard, K. E., & Quigley, B. M. (1999). Drinking and marital aggression in newlyweds: An event-based analysis of drinking and the occurrence of husband marital aggression. *Journal of Studies on Alcohol, 60*, 537–545.

Lessard v. Schmidt, 349 F. Supp 1078 E. D. Wis (1972).

Levensky, E. R., & Fruzzetti, A. E. (2003). Partner violence: Assessment, prediction, and intervention. In W. T. O'Donohue & E. R. Levensky (Eds.), *Handbook of forensic psychology* (pp. 713–741). New York: Elsevier Science.

Levenson, J. S. (2004). Sexual predator civil commitment: A comparison of selected and released offenders. *International Journal of Offender Therapy and Comparative Criminology, 48*, 638–648.

Levenson, J. S., & Cotter, L. P. (2005). The impact of sex offender residence restrictions: 1,000 feet from danger or one step from absurd. *International Journal of Offender Therapy and Comparative Criminology, 49*, 168–178.

Levenson, M. R., Kiehl, K. A., & Fitzpatrick, C. M. (1999). Assessing psychopathic in a noninstitutionalized population. *Journal of Personality and Social Psychology*, *68*, 151–158.

Levenston, G. K., Patrick, C. J., Bradley, M. M., & Lang, P. J. (2000). The psychopath as observers: Emotion and attention in picture processing. *Journal of Abnormal Psychology*, *109*, 373–385.

Levin, S. M., & Stava, L. (1987). Personality characteristics of sex offenders: A review. *Archives of Sexual Behavior*, *16*, 57–79.

Lidz, C. W. (1998). Coercion in psychiatric care: What have we learned from research? *Journal of the American Academy of Psychiatry and Law*, *26*, 631–637.

Lidz, C. W., Hoge, S. K., Gardner, W., Bennett, N. S., Monahan, J., Mulvey, E. P., et al. (1995). Perceived coercion in mental hospital admission: Pressures and process. *Archives of General Psychiatry*, *52*, 1034–1039.

Lidz, C. W., Mulvey, E. P., & Gardner, W. (1993). The accuracy of predictions of violence to others. *Journal of the American Medical Association*, *269*, 1007–1011.

Lidz, C. W., Mulvey, E. P., Hoge, S. K., Kirsch, B. L., Monahan, J., Bennett, N. S., et al. (1997). The validity of mental patients' accounts of coercion-related behaviors in the hospital admission process. *Law and Human Behavior*, *21*, 361–376.

Lidz, C. W., Mulvey, E. P., Hoge, S. K., Kirsch, B. L., Monahan, J., Eisenberg, M., et al. (1998). Factual sources of psychiatric patients' perceptions of coercion in the hospital admission process. *American Journal of Psychiatry*, *159*, 1254–1260.

Lidz, C. W., Mulvey, E. P., Hoge, S. K., Kirsch, B. L., Monahan, J., Bennett, N. S., et al. (2000). Sources of coercive behaviours in psychiatric admissions. *Acta Psychiatrica Scandinavica*, *101*, 73–79.

Lilienfeld, S. O. (1992). The association between antisocial personality and somatization disorders: A review and integration of theoretical models. *Clinical Psychology Review*, *12*, 641–662.

Lilienfeld, S. O., & Hess, T. H. (2001). Psychopathic personality traits and somatization: Sex differences in the mediating role of negative emotionality. *Journal of Psychopathology and Behavioral Assessment*, *23*, 11–24.

Lilienfeld, S. O., Lynn, S. J., & Lohr, J. M. (2003). *Science and pseudoscience in clinical psychology*. New York: Guilford Press.

Link, B. G., Monahan, J., Stueve, A., & Cullen, F. T. (1999). Real in their consequences: A sociological approach to understanding the association between psychotic symptoms and violence. *American Sociological Review*, *64*, 316–332.

Link, B. G., & Stueve, A. (1994). Psychotic symptoms and the violent/illegal behavior of mental patients compared to community controls. In J. Monahan & H. J. Steadman (Eds.), *Violence and mental disorder: Developments in risk assessment* (pp. 137–159). Chicago: University of Chicago Press.

Linton, S. J., Vlaeyen, J., & Ostelo, R. (2002). The back pain beliefs of health care providers: Are we fear avoidant? *Journal of Occupational Rehabilitation*, *12*, 223–232.

Lippel, K. (1999). Therapeutic and anti-therapeutic consequences of workers' compensation. *International Journal of Law and Psychiatry*, *22*, 521–546.

Lipsey, M. W. (1992). The effect of treatment on juvenile delinquents: Results from meta-analysis. In F. Lösel, D. Bender, & T. Bliesener (Eds.), *Psychology and law: International perspectives* (pp. 131–143). Oxford: Walter De Gruyter.

Lipsey, M. W., & Derzon, J. H. (1998). Predictors of violent or serious delinquency in adolescence and early adulthood: A synthesis of longitudinal research. In R.

Mittenberg, W., Patton, C., Canyock, E. M., & Condit, D. C. (2002). Base rates of malingering and symptom exaggeration. *Journal of Clinical and Experimental Neuropsychology, 24*, 1094–1102.

Mittenberg, W., Tremont, G., & Rayls, K. R. (1996). Impact of cognitive function on MMPI-2 validity in neurologically impaired patients. *Assessment, 3*, 157–163.

M'Naghten's Case, 8 Eng. Rep 718 (1843).

Mobley, M. J. (1999). Psychotherapy with criminal offenders. In I. B. Weiner & A. K. Hess (Eds.), *Handbook for forensic psychology* (2nd ed., pp. 603–639). Hoboken, NJ: John Wiley & Sons.

Mobley, M. J. (2006). Psychotherapy with criminal offenders. In I. B. Weiner & A. K. Hess (Eds.), *Handbook for forensic psychology* (3rd ed., pp. 751–789). Hoboken, NJ: John Wiley & Sons.

Moffitt, T. E. (1993). Adolescence-limited and life-course-persistent antisocial behavior: A developmental taxonomy. *Psychological Review, 100*, 674–701.

Moffitt, T. E. (2006). Life-course-persistent versus adolescence-limited antisocial behavior. In D. Cicchetti & D. J. Cohen (Eds.), *Developmental psychopathology: Vol. 3. Risk, disorder, and adaptation* (2nd ed., pp. 570–598). Hoboken, NJ: John Wiley & Sons.

Monahan, J. (1981). *The clinical prediction of violent behavior*. Rockville, MD, NIMH.

Monahan, J. (1984). The prediction of violent behavior: Toward a second generation of theory and policy. *American Journal of Psychiatry, 141*, 10–15.

Monahan, J. (1988). Risk assessment of violence among the mentally disordered: Generating useful knowledge. *International Journal of Law and Psychiatry, 11*, 249–257.

Monahan, J. (1992). Risk assessment: Commentary on Poythress and Otto. *Forensic Reports, 5*, 151–154.

Monahan, J. (1996). Violence prediction: The past twenty and the next twenty years. *Criminal Justice and Behavior, 23*, 107–120.

Monahan, J. (2002). The MacArthur studies of violence risk. *Criminal Behaviour and Mental Health, 12*, 67–72.

Monahan, J. (2003). Violence risk assessment. In A. M. Goldstein (Ed.), *Handbook of psychology: Vol. 11. Forensic psychology* (pp. 527–540). Hoboken, NJ: John Wiley & Sons.

Monahan, J., & Arnold, J. (1996). Violence by people with mental illness: A consensus statement by advocates and researchers. *Psychiatric Rehabilitation Journal, 19*, 67–70.

Monahan, J., Heilbrun, K., Silver, E., Nabors, E., Bone, J., & Slovic, P. (2002). Frequency formats, vivid outcomes, and forensic settings. *International Journal of Forensic Mental Health, 1*, 121–126.

Monahan, J., & Shah, S. A. (1989). Dangerousness and commitment of the mentally disordered in the United States. *Schizophrenia Bulletin, 15*, 541–553.

Monahan, J., & Silver, E. (2003). Judicial decision thresholds for violence risk management. *International Journal of Forensic Mental Health, 2*, 1–6.

Monahan, J., & Steadman, H. J. (1996). Violent storms and violent people: How meteorology can inform risk communication in mental health law. *American Psychologist, 51*, 931–938.

Monahan, J., & Steadman, H. L. (1994). *Violence and mental disorder: Developments in risk assessment*. Chicago: The University of Chicago Press.

Monahan, J., Steadman, H. J., Robbins, P. C., Appelbaum, P., Banks, S., Grisso, T., et al. (2005). An actuarial model of violence risk assessment for persons with mental disorders. *Psychiatric Services*, *56*, 810–815.

Monahan, J., Steadman, H. J., Silver, E., Appelbaum, P. S., Robbins, P. C., Mulvey, E. P., et al. (2001). *Rethinking risk assessment: The MacArthur study of mental disorder and violence*. New York: Oxford University Press.

Monahan, J., & Walker, L. (1980). Social science research in law: A new paradigm. *American Psychologist*, *43*, 465–472.

Monson, C. M., Gunnin, D. D., Fogel, M. H., & Kyle, L. (2001). Stopping (or slowing) the revolving door: Factors related to NGRI acquittees' maintenance of a conditional release. *Law and Human Behavior*, *25*, 257–267.

Montross, L. P., Zisook, S., & Kasckow, J. (2005). Suicide among patients with schizophrenia: A consideration of risk and protective factors. *Annals of Clinical Psychiatry*, *17*, 173–182.

Moran, R. (1981). *Knowing right from wrong: The insanity defense of Daniel McNaughtan*. New York: The Free Press.

Moriarity, J. C. (2001). Wonders of the invisible world: Prosecutorial syndrome and profile evidence in the Salem Witchcraft trials. *Vermont Law Review*, *26*, 43–99.

Mossman, D. (1994). Assessing predictions of violence: Being accurate about accuracy. *Journal of Consulting and Clinical Psychology*, *62*, 783–792.

Mossman, D. (1999). "Hired guns," "whores," and "prostitutes": Case law references to clinicians of ill repute. *Journal of the American Academy of Psychiatry and the Law*, *27*, 414–425.

Mossman, D., & Kapp, M. B. (1998). "Courtoom whores"? – or why do attorneys call us?: Findings from a survey on attorneys' use of mental health experts. *Journal of the American Academy of Psychiatry and the Law*, *26*, 27–36.

Moye, J. (2003). Guardianship and conservatorhsip. In T. Grisso (Ed.) *Evaluating competencies: Forensic assessments and instruments* (pp. 309–389). New York: Kluwer Academic/Plenum Publishers.

Mumley, D. L., Tillbrook, C. E., & Grisso, T. (2003). Five year research update (1996–2000): Evaluations for competence to stand trial (adjudicative competence). *Behavioral Sciences and the Law*, *21*, 329–350.

Munsterberg, H. (1908). *On the witness stand*. New York: Doubleday, Page, and Company.

Murphy, C. M., & Cascardi, M. (1993). Psychological aggression and abuse in marriage. In R. L. Hampton, T. P. Gollotta, G. R. Adams, E. H. Potter, & R. P. Weissberg (Eds.), *Family violence: Prevention and treatment* (pp. 86–112). Newbury Park, CA: Sage.

Murrie, D. C., & Warren, J. I. (2005). Clinician variation in rates of legal sanity opinions: Implications for self-monitoring. *Professional Psychology: Research and Practice*, *36*, 519–524.

Myers, B., & Arena, M. P. (2001). Trial consultation: A new direction in applied psychology. *Professional Psychology: Research and Practice*, *32*, 386–391.

National Adolescent Perpetrator Network. (1993). The revised report from the National Task Force on Juvenile Sex Offending. *Juvenile and Family Court Journal*, *44*, 1–120.

National School Safety Center (2003). School associated violent deaths. Westlake Village, CA. Retrieved March 17, 2007 from http://www.schoolsafety.us/School-Associated-Violent-Deaths-p-6.html

Nebraska Revised Statutes § 28-311.03 (Cum. Supp. 2004).

Newman, J. P. (1998). Psychopathic behavior: An information processing perspective. In D. J. Cooke, R. D. Hare, & A. Forth (Eds.), *Psychopathy: Theory, research and implications for society* (pp. 81–104). The Netherlands: Kluwer Academic Publishers.

Newman, J. P., MacCoon, D. G., Vaughn, L. J., & Sadeh, N. (2005). Validating a distinction between primary and secondary psychopathy with measures of Gray's BIS and BAS constructs. *Journal of Abnormal Psychology, 114,* 319–323.

Newman, J. P., Schmitt, W. A., & Voss, W. D. (1997). The impact of motivationally neutral cues on psychopathic individuals: Assessing the generality of the response modulation hypothesis. *Journal of Abnormal Psychology, 106,* 563–575.

Nicholls, T. L., Ogloff, J. R. P., & Douglas, K. S. (2004). Assessing risk for violence among male and female civil psychiatric patients: The HCR-20, PCL: SV, and VSC. *Behavioral Sciences & the Law, 22,* 127–158.

Nichols, H. R., & Molinder, I. (1996). *Multiphasic sexual inventory II handbook.* Tacoma, WA: Nichols & Molinder Associates.

Nicholson, R. A. (1999). Forensic assessment. In R. Roesch, S. Hart, & J. R. P. Ogloff (Eds.), *Psychology and the law: State of the discipline* (pp. 121–167). Dordrecht, The Netherlands: Kluwer Academic/Plenum Publishers.

Nicholson, R. A., Barnard, G. W., Robbins, L., & Hankins, G. (1994). Predicting treatment outcome for incompetent defendants. *Bulletin of the American Academy of Psychiatry and Law, 22,* 367–377.

Nicholson, R. A., Briggs, S. R., & Robertson, H. C. (1988). Instruments for assessing competency to stand trial: How do they work? *Professional Psychology: Research and Practice, 19,* 383–394.

Nicholson, R. A., Ekenstam, C., & Norwood, S. (1996). Coercion and the outcome of psychiatric hospitalization. *International Journal of Law and Psychiatry, 19,* 201–217.

Nicholson, R. A., & Kugler, K. E. (1991). Competent and incompetent criminal defendants: A quantitative review of comparison research. *Psychological Bulletin, 109,* 355–370.

Nicholson, R. A., & McNulty, J. L. (1992). Outcome of hospitalization for defendants found incompetent to stand trial. *Behavioral Sciences & the Law, 10,* 371–383.

Nicholson, R. A., & Norwood, S. (2000). The quality of forensic psychological assessments, reports, and testimony: Acknowledging the gap between promise and practice. *Law and Human Behavior, 24,* 9–44.

Nicholson, R. A., Norwood, S., & Enyart, C. (1991). Characteristics and outcomes of insanity acquittees in Oklahoma. *Behavioral Sciences and the Law, 9,* 487–500.

Nicholson, R. A., Robertson, H. C., Johnson, W. G., & Jensen, G. (1988). A comparison of instruments for assessing competency to stand trial. *Law and Human Behavior, 12,* 313–321.

Nietzel, M. T., McCarthy, D. M., & Kern, M. J. (1999). The current state of the empirical literature. In R. Roesch, S. Hart, & J. R. P. Ogloff (Eds.), *Psychology and the law: State of the discipline* (pp. 25–52). Dordrecht, The Netherlands: Kluwer Academic/Plenum Publishers.

Norris, D. M. (2003). Forensic consultation and the clergy sexual abuse crisis. *Journal of the American Academy of Psychiatry and the Law, 31,* 154–157.

Nusbaum, D. J. (2002). The craziest reform of them all: A critical analysis of the constitutional implications of "abolishing the insanity defense." *Cornell Law Review, 87,* 1509–1571.

O'Brien, B. S., & Frick, P. J. (1996). Reward dominance: Associations with anxiety, conduct problems, and psychopathy in children. *Journal of Abnormal Child Psychology, 24,* 223–240.

O'Brien, M., Mortimer, L., Singleton, N., Meltzer, H., & Goodman, R. (2003). Psychiatric morbidity among women prisoners in England and Wales. *International Review of Psychiatry, 15,* 153–157.

O'Connor v. Donaldson, 422 U.S. 563 (1975).

O'Donohue, W., Letourneau, E., & Dowling, H. (1997). Development and preliminary validation of a paraphilic sexual fantasy questionnaire. *Sexual Abuse: A Journal of Research and Treatment, 9,* 167–78.

O'Farrell, T. J., Fals-Stewart, W., Murphy, M., & Murphy, C. M. (2003). Partner violence before and after individually based alcoholism treatment for male alcoholic patients. *Journal of Consulting and Clinical Psychology, 71,* 92–102.

Ogloff, J. R. P. (1991). A comparison of insanity defense standards on juror decision making. *Law and Human Behavior, 15,* 509–531.

Ogloff, J. R. P. (1999). Ethical and legal contours of forensic psychology. In R. Roesch, S. Hart, & J. R. P. Ogloff (Eds.), *Psychology and the law: State of the discipline* (pp. 405–422). Dordrecht, The Netherlands: Kluwer Academic/Plenum Publishers.

Ogloff, J. R. P. (2002). Identifying and accommodating the needs of the mentally ill people in gaols and prisons. *Psychiatry, Psychology, and Law, 9,* 1–33.

Ogloff, J. R. P. (2004). Invited introductory remarks to the special issue. *Canadian Journal of Behavioural Sciences, 36,* 84–86.

Ogloff, J. R. P., & Cronshaw, S. F. (2001). Expert psychological testimony: Assisting or misleading the trier of fact? *Canadian Psychology, 42,* 87–91.

Ogloff, J. R. P., & Finkelman, D. (1999). Psychology and law: An overview. In R. Roesch, S. D. Hart, & J. R. P. Ogloff (Eds.), *Psychology and law: The state of the discipline* (pp. 1–20). Dordrecht, Netherlands: Kluwer Academic Publishers.

Ogloff, J. R. P., & Rose, V. G. (2005). The comprehension of judicial instructions. In N. Brewer and K. D. Williams (Eds.), *Psychology and law: An empirical perspective* (pp. 407–444). New York: Guilford Press.

Ogloff, J. R. P., Wong, S., & Greenwood, A. (1990). Treating criminal psychopaths in a therapeutic community program. *Behavioral Sciences and the Law, 8,* 81–90.

O'Leary, K. D. (1999). Psychological abuse: A variable deserving critical attention in domestic violence. *Violence and Victims, 14,* 3–23.

O'Leary, K. D., & Curley, A. (1985). Assertion training for abused wives: A potentially hazardous treatment. *Journal of Marital & Family Therapy, 1,* 319–322.

O'Leary, K. D., Heyman, R. E., & Jongsma, A. E. (1998). *The couples psychotherapy treatment planner.* Hoboken, NJ: John Wiley & Sons, Inc.

O'Leary, K. D., Malone, J., & Tyree, A. (1994). Physical aggression in early marriage: Prerelationship and relationship effects. *Journal of Consulting and Clinical Psychology, 62,* 594–602.

O'Leary, K. D., Vivian, D., & Malone, J. (1992). Assessment of physical aggression against women in marriage: The need for multimodal assessment. *Behavioral Assessment, 14,* 5–14.

O'Leary, K. D., & Woodin, E. M. (2006). Bringing the agendas together: Partner and child abuse. In J. R. Lutzker (Ed.), *Preventing violence: Research and evidence-based intervention strategies* (pp. 239–258). Washington, DC: American Psychological Association.

Olmstead v. L. C., 527 U.S. 581 (1999).

Ostrom, B. J., Kauder, N. B., & LaFountain, R. C. (2001). *Examining the work of state courts, 2001.* Williamsburg, VA: National Center for State Courts.

O'Toole, M. E. (2000). *The school shooter: A threat assessment perspective.* Quantico, VA: Federal Bureau of Investigation, National Center for the Analysis of Violent Crime.

Otto, R. K. (1989). Bias and expert testimony of mental health professionals in adversarial proceedings: A preliminary investigation. *Behavioral Sciences and the Law, 7,* 267–273.

Otto, R. K. (1992). Prediction of dangerous behavior: A review and analysis of "second generation" research. *Forensic Reports, 5,* 103–133.

Otto, R., & Borum, R. (2003). Evaluation of youth in the juvenile justice system. In W. T. O'Donohue & E. R. Levensky (Eds.), *Handbook of forensic psychology: Resource for mental health and legal professionals* (pp. 873–895). New York: Elsevier Science.

Otto, R. K., Buffington-Vollum, J. K., & Edens, J. F. (2003). Child custody evaluation. In A. M. Goldstein (Ed.), *Handbook of psychology: Vol. 11. Forensic psychology* (pp. 179–208). New York: John Wiley & Sons, Inc.

Otto, R. K., Edens, J. F., & Barcus, E. H. (2000). The use of psychological testing in child custody evaluations. *Family and Conciliation Courts Review, 38,* 312–340.

Otto, R. K., & Heilbrun, K. (2002). The practice of forensic psychology: A look toward the future in the light of the past. *American Psychologist, 57,* 5–18.

Packer, I. K., & Borum, R. (2003). Forensic training in practice. In A. M. Goldstein (Ed.), *Handbook of psychology: Vol. 11. Forensic psychology* (pp. 21–32). Hoboken, NJ: John Wiley & Sons, Inc.

Palarea, R. E., Zona, M. A., Lane, J. C., & Langhinrichsen-Rohling, J. (1999). The dangerous nature of intimate relationship stalking: Threats, violence, and associated risk factors. *Behavioral Sciences and the Law, 17,* 269–283.

Palmore v. Sidoti, 466 U.S. 429, 104 S. Ct. 1879, 80 L. Ed. 2d 421 (1984).

Parker, R. S. (2001). *Concussive brain trauma: Neurobehavioral impairment and maladaption.* London: CRC Press.

Pasewark, R. A., & McGinley, H. (1985). Insanity plea: National survey of frequency and success. *Journal of Psychiatry & Law, 13,* 101–108.

Pasewark, R. A., Pantle, M. L., & Steadman, H. J. (1982). Detention and rearrest rates of persons found not guilty by reason of insanity and convicted felons. *American Journal of Psychiatry, 139,* 892–897.

Pastors, M. C., Moltó, J., Vila, J., & Lang, P. J. (2003). Startle reflex modulation, affective ratings and autonomic reactivity in incarcerated Spanish psychopaths. *Psychophysiology, 40,* 934–938.

Pate v. Robinson, 383 U.S. 375 (1966).

Paterson, B. (2006). Newspaper representations of mental illness and the impact of the reporting of "events" on social policy: The "framing" of Isabel Schawartz and Jonathan Zito. *Journal of Psychiatric and Mental Health Nursing, 13,* 294–300.

Patrick, C. (1994). Emotion and psychopathy: Startling new insights. *Psychophysiology, 31,* 319–330.

Patry, M. W., Stinson, V., & Smith, S. M. (2008). CSI effect: Is popular television transforming Canadian society? In J. Greenberg & C. Elliott (Eds.), *Communications in question: Canadian perspectives on controversial issues in communication studies* (pp. 291–298). Scarborough, Ontario: Thompson-Nelson.

Patterson, C. M., & Newman, J. P. (1993). Reflectivity and learning from aversive events: Toward a psychological mechanism for the syndromes of disinhibition. *Psychological Review, 100,* 716–738.

Penrod, S. D., & Cutler, B. L. (1987). Assessing the competencies of juries. In I. B. Weiner & A. K. Hess (Eds.), *Handbook for forensic psychology* (pp. 293–318). New York: John Wiley & Sons.

People v. McQuillan, 392 Mich. 511, 221 N.W.2d 569 (1974).

People v. Wells 33 Cal.2d 330 (1949).

Perlin, M. L. (2003). Therapeutic jurisprudence and outpatient commitment law: Kendra's law as a case study. *Psychology, Public Policy, and the Law, 9,* 183–208.

Perlin, M. (1996). Myths, realities, and the political world: The anthropology of insanity defense attitudes. *Bulletin of the American Academy of Psychiatry and the Law, 24,* 5–26.

Perlin, M. L. (1992). Fatal assumption: A critical evaluation of the role of counsel in mental disability cases. *Law and Human Behavior, 16,* 39–59.

Peruzzi, N., & Bongar, B. (1999). Assessing risk for completed suicide in patients with major depression: Psychologists' views of critical factors. *Professional Psychology: Research and Practice, 30,* 576–580.

Petrella, R. C., & Poythress, N. G. (1983). The quality of forensic evaluations: An interdisciplinary study. *Journal of Consulting and Clinical Psychology, 51,* 76–85.

Pham, T. H., Vanderstukken, O., Philippot, P., & Vanderlinden, M. (2003). Selective attention and executive functions deficits among criminal psychopaths. *Aggressive Behavior, 29,* 393–405.

Pincus, T. (2005). Effect of cognition on pain experiences and pain behavior: Diathesis-stress and the casual conundrum. In G. Young, A. W. Kane, & K. Nicholson (Eds.), *Psychological knowledge in court: PTSD, pain, and TBI* (pp. 163–180). New York: Springer.

Pinta, E. R. (2001). The prevalence of serious mental disorders among U.S. prisoners. In G. Landsberg & A. Smiley (Eds.), *Forensic mental health: Working with offenders with mental illness* (pp. 12-1–12-10). Kingston, NJ: Civic Research Institute.

Pithers, W. D., Marques, J. K., Gibat, C. C., & Marlatt, G. A. (1983). Relapse prevention with sexual aggressives: A self-control model of treatment and maintenance of change. In J. C. Greer & I. R. Stuart (Eds.), *The sexual aggressor: Current perspectives on treatment* (pp. 214–239). New York: Van Nostrand Reinhold.

Plante, T. G. (2003). Priests behaving badly: What do we know about priest sex offenders? *Sexual Addiction and Compulsivity, 9,* 93–97.

Platt, A. M., & Diamond, B. L. (1965). The origins and development of the "wild beast" concept of mental illness and its relation to theories of criminal responsibility. *Journal of the History of the Behavioral Sciences, 1,* 355–367.

Pokorny, A. (1983). Prediction of suicide in psychiatric patients: Report of a prospective study. *Archives of General Psychiatry, 40,* 249–257.

Pollock, A. L., & Webster, B. D. (1993). Psychology and the law: The emerging role of forensic psychology. In K. S. Dobson & D. J. Dobson (Eds.), *Professional psychology in Canada* (pp. 391–412). Ashland, OH: Hogrefe & Huber Publishers.

Porter, S., Campbell, M. A., Woodworth, M., & Birt, A. R. (2001). A new psychological conceptualization of the sexual psychopath. In F. Columbus (Ed.), *Advances in psychology research* (Vol. 7, pp. 21–36). Hauppauge, NY: Nova Science Publishers, Inc.

Porter, S., Campbell, M. A., Woodworth, M., & Birt, A. R. (2002). A new psychological conceptualization of the sexual psychopath. In S. P. Shohov (Ed.), *Advances in psychology research* (Vol. 15, pp. 51–65). Hauppauge, NY: Nova Science Publishers, Inc.

Porter, S., Fairweather, D., Drugge, J., Hervé, H., & Birt, A. (2000). Profiles of psychopathy in incarcerated sexual offenders. *Criminal Justice and Behavior, 27*, 216–233.

Porter, S., & Woodworth, M. (2006). Psychopathy and aggression. In C. J. Patrick (Ed.), *Handbook of psychopathy* (pp. 481–494). New York: Guilford Press.

Pothast, H. L., & Allen, C. M. (1994). Masculinity and femininity in male and female perpetrators of child sexual abuse. *Child Abuse & Neglect, 18*, 753–767.

Poulsen, H. D., & Engberg, M. (2001). Validation of psychiatric patients' statements on coercive measures. *Acta Psychiatrica Scandinavica, 103*, 60–65.

Poulson, R. L. (1990). Mock juror attribution of criminal responsibility: Effects of race and the guilty but mentally ill (GBMI) verdict option. *Journal of Applied Social Psychology, 20*, 1596–1611.

Poulson, R. L., Braithwaite, R. L., Brondino, M. J., & Wuensch, K. L. (1997). Mock jurors' insanity defense verdict selections: The role of evidence, attitudes, and verdict options. *Journal of Social Behavior and Personality, 12*, 743–758.

Poulson, R. L., Wuensch, K. L., & Brondino, M. J. (1998). Factors that discriminate among mock jurors' verdict selections: Impact of the guilty but mentally ill verdict option. *Criminal Justice and Behavior, 25*, 366–381.

Poythress, N. G. (1992). Expert testimony on violence and dangerousness: Roles for mental health professionals. *Forensic Reports, 5*, 134–150.

Poythress, N. G., Bonnie, R. J., Hoge, S. K., Monahan, J., & Oberlander, L. B. (1994) Client abilities to assist counsel and make decisions in criminal cases: Findings from three studies. *Law and Human Behavior, 18*, 437–452.

Poythress, N., Melton, G. B., Petrila, J., & Slobogin, C. (2000). Commentary on "the Mental State at the Time of the Offense Measure". *Journal of the American Academy of Psychiatry and the Law, 28*, 29–32.

Poythress, N. G., Nicholson, R., Otto, R. K., Edens, J. F., Bonnie, R. J., Monahan, J., et al. (1999). *The MacArthur Competence Assessment Tool-Criminal Adjudication: Professional manual*. Odessa, FL: Psychological Assessment Resources, Inc.

Pulliam v. Smith, 348 N.C. 616, 501 S.E.2d 898 (1998).

Prentky, R., Harris, B., Frizzell, K., & Righthand, S. (2000). An actuarial procedure for assessing risk with juvenile sex offenders. *Sexual Abuse: A Journal of Research and Treatment, 12*, 71–94.

Quinsey, V. L., Harris, G. T., Rice, M. E., & Cormier, C. A. (1998). *Violent offenders: Appraising and managing risk*. Washington, DC: American Psychological Association.

Quinsey, V. L., Harris, G. T., Rice, M. E., & Cormier, C. A. (2006). *Violent offenders: Appraising and managing risk* (2nd ed.). Washington, DC: American Psychological Association.

Quinsey, V. L., Rice, M. E., & Harris, G. T. (1995). Actuarial prediction of sexual recidivism. *Journal of Interpersonal Violence, 10*, 85–105.

Raeder, M. S. (1997). The better way: The role of batterers' profiles and expert "social framework" background in cases implicating domestic violence. *University of Colorado Law Review, 68*, 147–207.

Rand, M., & Strom, K. (1997). *Violence-related injuries treated in hospital emergency departments* (NCJ 156921). Washington, DC: U.S. Department of Justice.

Randazzo, M. R., Borum, R., Vossekuil, B., Fein, R., Modzlelski, W., & Pollack, W. (2006). Threat assessment in schools: Empirical support and comparison with other approaches. In S. R. Jimerson & M. Furlong (Eds.), *Handbook of school violence and school safety: From research to practice* (pp. 147–156). Mahwah, NJ: Lawrence Erlbaum Associates Publishers.

Rapp, L. A., & Wodarski, J. S. (1997). Juvenile violence: The high risk factors, current interventions, and implications for social work practice. *Journal of Applied Social Sciences*, *22*, 3–14.

Redding, R. E., Floyd, M. Y., & Hawk, G. L. (2001). What judges and lawyers think about the testimony of mental health experts: A survey of the courts and bar. *Behavioral Sciences and the Law*, *19*, 583–594.

Redding, R. E., Goldstein, N. E. S., & Heilbrun, K. (2005). Juvenile delinquency: Past and present. In K. Heilbrun, N. E. S. Goldstein, & R. E. Redding, *Juvenile delinquency: Prevention, assessment, and intervention* (pp. 3–18). New York: Oxford University Press.

Reed, J. (1996). Editorial: Psychopathy – A clinical and legal dilemma. *British Journal of Psychiatry*, *168*, 4–9.

Regina v. Lavelle, 65 C.R. (3d) 387 (1988).

Regina v. Mohan, 89 C.C.C. (3d) 402 (S.C.C.) (1994).

Regina v. Whittle, 2 S.C.R. 914 (1994).

Rennison, C. M. (2003). *Intimate partner violence, 1993–2001* (NCJ 197838). Washington, DC: U.S. Department of Justice.

Rex v. Arnold, 16 How. St. Tr. (1724).

Rice, M. E., & Harris, G. T. (1997). Cross-validation and extension of the Violence Risk Appraisal Guide for child molesters and rapists. *Law and Human Behavior*, *21*, 231–241.

Rice, M. E., & Harris, G. T. (1995). Violent recidivism: Assessing predictive validity. *Journal of Consulting and Clinical Psychology*, *63*, 737–748.

Rice, M. E., Harris, G. T., & Cormier, C. A. (1992). An evaluation of a maximum security therapeutic community for psychopaths and other mentally disordered offenders. *Law and Human Behavior*, *16*, 399–412.

Rice, M. E., Harris, G. T., & Quinsey, V. L. (1990). A follow-up of rapists assessed in a maximum-security psychiatric facility. *Journal of Interpersonal Violence*, *5*, 435–448.

Richardson, J. T., Ginsburg, G. P., Gatowski, S., & Dobbin, S. (1995). The problems associated with applying Daubert to psychological syndrome evidence. *Judicature*, *79*, 10–16.

Richman, J., Green, P., Gervais, R., Flaro, L., Merten, T., Brockhaus, R., et al. (2006). Objective tests of symptom exaggeration in independent medical examinations. *Journal of Occupational and Environmental Medicine*, *48*, 303–311.

Riggins v. Nevada, 112 S. Ct. 1810 (1992).

Riggs, D. S., Kilpatrick, D. G., & Resnick, H. S. (1992). Long-term psychological distress associated with marital rape and aggravated assault: A comparison to other crime victims. *Journal of Family Violence*, *7*, 283–296.

Righthand, S., Prentky, R., Knight, R., Carpenter, E., Hecker, J. E., & Nangle, D. (2005). Factor structure and validation of the Juvenile Sex Offender Assessment Protocol (J-SOAP). *Sexual Abuse: Journal of Research and Treatment*, *17*, 13–30.

Initial findings from a randomized controlled trial. *Research in Community Mental Health, 10,* 57–77.

Swartz, M. S., Swanson, J. W., & Hannon, M. J. (2003). Does fear of coercion keep people away from mental health treatment? Evidence from a survey of persons with schizophrenia and mental health professionals. *Behavioral Sciences & the Law, 21,* 459–472.

Swartz, M. S., Swanson, J. W., Hiday, V. A., Wagner, H. R., Burns, B. J., & Borum, R. (2001). A randomized controlled trial of out patient commitment in North Carolina. *Psychiatric Services, 52,* 325–329.

Tanenhaus, D. S. (2000). The evolution of transfer out of the juvenile court. In J. Fagan & F. E. Zimring (Eds.), *The changing borders of juvenile justice: Transfer of adolescents to the criminal court* (pp. 13–43). Chicago: University of Chicago Press.

Tarasoff v. Regents of the University of California, 17 Cal. 3d 425, 551 P.2d 334, 131 Cal. Rptr. 14 (Cal. 1976),

Tarolla, S. M., Wagner, E. F., Rabinowitz, J., & Tubman, J. G. (2002). Understanding and treating juvenile offenders: A review of current knowledge and future directions. *Aggression and Violent Behavior, 7,* 125–143.

Taslitz, A. E. (1995). Daubert guide to the Federal Rules of Evidence: A not-so-plain meaning. *Harvard Journal of Legislation, 32,* 3–35.

Taylor, J. S. (1999). The legal environment pertaining to clinical neuropsychology. In J. J. Sweet (Ed.), *Forensics Neuropsychology* (pp. 419–442). Lisse, The Netherlands: Swets & Zeitlinger.

Tengström, A., Grann, M., Långström, N., & Kullgren, G. (2000). Psychopathy (PCL-R) as a predictor of violent recidivism among criminal offenders with schizophrenia. *Law and Human Behavior, 24,* 45–58.

Teplin, L. A. (1983). The criminalization of the mentally ill: Speculation in search of data. *Psychological Bulletin, 94,* 54–67.

Teplin, L. A. (1984). Criminalizing mental disorder: The comparative arrest rate of the mentally ill. *American Psychologist, 39,* 794–803.

Teplin, L. A. (2001). Police discretion and mentally ill persons. In G. Landsberg & A. Smiley (Eds.), *Forensic mental health: Working with offenders with mental illness* (pp. 28-1–28-11). Kingston, NJ: Civic Research Institute.

Teplin, L. A., McClelland, G. M., Abram, K. M., & Weiner, D. A. (2005). Crime victimization in adults with severe mental illness: Comparison with the National Crime Victimization. *Archives of General Psychiatry, 62,* 911–921.

Thompson, M. P., & Kingree, J. B. (2006). The roles of victim and perpetrator alcohol use in intimate partner violence outcomes. *Journal of Interpersonal Violence, 21,* 163–177.

Thor, P. (1993). Finding incompetency in guardianship: Standardizing the process. *Arizona Law Review, 35,* 739–764.

Timmons-Mitchell, J., Bender, M. B., Kishna, M. A., & Mitchell, C. C. (2006). An independent effectiveness trial of multisystemic therapy with juvenile justice youth. *Journal of Clinical Child and Adolescent Psychology, 35,* 227–236.

Tjaden P., & Thoeness, N. (1998). *Stalking in America: Findings from the National Violence Against Women Survey.* Washington, DC: National Institute of Justice, U.S. Department of Justice.

Torres, A. N., Boccaccini, M. T., & Miller, H. A. (2006). Perceptions of the validity and utility of criminal profiling among forensic psychologists and psychiatrists. *Professional Psychology Research and Practice, 37,* 51–58.

Turkheimer, E., & Parry, C. D. (1992). Why the gap? Practice and policy in civil commitment hearings. *American Psychologist, 47,* 646–655.

Tyler, T. R. (2006). Restorative justice and procedural justice: Dealing with rule breaking. *Journal of Social Issues, 62,* 307–326.

Tyler, J., Darville, R., & Stalnaker, K. (2001). Juvenile boot camps: A descriptive analysis of program diversity and effectiveness. *Social Science Journal, 38,* 445–460.

United States v. Brawner, 471 F. 2d 969 (D.C. Cir. 1972).

United States v. Hinckley, 525 F. Supp. 1342 (D. D.C. 1981).

U.S. Department of Health and Human Services, National Center on Child Abuse and Neglect. (1995). *Child maltreatment 1993: Reports from the States to the National Center on Child Abuse and Neglect.* Washington, DC: US Government Printing Office.

U.S. Department of Justice. (1999). *Women offenders.* NCJ 175688. Washington, DC: Bureau of Justice Statistics.

U.S. Department of Justice. (2001). *Office of Juvenile Justice and Delinquency Prevention research 2000.* Washington, DC: Author.

U.S. Department of Justice. (2002). *Uniform crime report: 2001.* Washington, DC: Government Printing Office.

U.S. Surgeon General. (2001). *Youth violence: A report of the Surgeon General.* Rockville, MD: U.S. Dept. of Health and Human Services.

Vandiver, D. M., & Teske, R. (2006). Juvenile female and male sex offenders: A comparison of offender, victim, and judicial processing characteristics. *International Journal of Offender Therapy and Comparative Criminology, 50,* 148–165.

Van Dorsten, B. (2002). Forensic psychology. In B. Van Dorsten (Ed.), *Forensic psychology: From classroom to courtroom* (pp. 1–16). New York: Kluwer/Plenum.

Van Dorsten, B., & James, L. B. (2002). Forensic medical psychology. In B. Van Dorsten (Ed.), *Forensic psychology: From classroom to courtroom.* New York: Kluwer Academic/Plenum Publishers.

Vasquez, M. J. T., Baker, N. L., & Shullman, S. L. (2003). Assessing employment discrimination and harassment. In A. M. Goldstein (Ed.), *Handbook of psychology: Vol. 11. Forensic psychology* (pp. 259–277). New York: John Wiley & Sons, Inc.

Verger, D. M. (1992). The making of the insanity plea. *American Journal of Forensic Psychology, 10,* 35–47.

Verona, E., & Vitale, J. (2006). Psychopathy in women: Assessment, manifestations, and etiology. In C. J. Patrick (Ed.), *Handbook of psychopathy* (pp. 415–436). New York: Guilford Press.

Victor, T. L., & Abeles, N. (2004). Coaching clients to take psychological and neuro-psychological tests: A clash of ethical obligations. *Professional Psychology: Research and Practice, 35,* 373–379.

Viljoen, J. I., Roesch, R., Ogloff, J. R. P., & Zapf, P. A. (2003). The role of Canadian psychologists in conducting fitness and criminal responsibility evaluations. *Canadian Psychology, 44,* 369–381.

Viljoen, J. L., Roesch, R., & Zapf, P. A. (2002). Interrater reliability of the Fitness Interview Test across 4 professional groups. *Canadian Journal of Psychiatry, 47,* 945–952.

Vitale, J. E., & Newman, J. P. (2001). Using the Psychopathy Checklist-Revised with female samples: Reliability, validity, and implications for clinical utility. *Clinical Psychology: Science and Practice, 8,* 117–132.

Vitale, J. E., Newman, J. P., Bates, J. E., Goodnight, J., Dodge, K. A., & Pettit, G. S. (2005). Deficient behavioral inhibition and anomalous selective attention in a community sample of adolescents with psychopathic traits and low-anxiety traits. *Journal of Abnormal Child Psychology, 33*, 461–470.

Vitale, J. E., Smith, S. S., Brinkley, C. A., & Newman, J. P. (2002). The reliability and validity of the Psychopathy Checklist-Revised in a sample of female offenders. *Criminal Justice and Behavior, 29*, 202–231.

Vivian, D. & Langhinrichsen-Rohling, J. (1994). Are bi-directionality violent couples mutually victimized? A gender-sensitive comparison. *Violence and Victims, 9*, 107–124.

Vore, D. A. (2007). The disability psychological independent medical evaluation: Case law, ethical issues, and procedures. In A. M. Goldstein (Ed.), *Forensic psychology: Emerging topics and expanding roles* (pp. 489–510). Hoboken, NJ: John Wiley & Sons.

Waite, D., Keller, A., McGarvey, E. L., Wieckowski, E., Pinkerton, R., & Brown, G. (2005). Juvenile sex offender re-arrest rates for sexual, violent nonsexual, and property cirimes: A 10-year follow-up. *Sexual Abuse: A Journal of Research and Treatment, 17*, 313–331.

Walfish, S. (2006). Conducting personal injury evaluations. In I. B. Weiner & A. K. Hess (Eds.), *The handbook of forensic psychology* (pp. 124–139). Hoboken, NJ: John Wiley & Sons.

Walker, L. E. (1979). *The battered woman.* New York: Harper and Row.

Walker, L. E. (1984). *The battered woman syndrome.* New York: Springer.

Wallace, J. F., Vitale, J. E., & Newman, J. P. (1999). Response modulation deficits: Implications for the diagnosis and treatment of psychopathy. *Journal of Cognitive Psychotherapy, 13*, 55–70.

Waller, E. M., & Daniel, A. E. (2005). Purpose and utility of child custody evaluations: Attorney's perspective. *Journal of the American Academy of Psychiatry and the Law, 33*, 199–207.

Wallerstein, J. S., & Blakeslee, S. (1989). *Second chances: Men, women, and children a decade after divorce.* New York: Ticknor & Fields.

Walters, G. D. (2003a). Changes in outcome expectancies and criminal thinking following a brief course of psychoeducation. *Personality and Individual Differences, 35*, 691–701.

Walters, G. D. (2003b). Predicting criminal justice outcomes with the psychopathy checklist and lifestyle criminality screening form: A meta-analytic comparison. *Behavioral Sciences and the Law, 21*, 89–102.

Wardell, L., Gillespie, D. L., & Leffler, L. (1983). Science and violence against wives. In D. Finkelhor, R. J. Gelles, G. T. Hotaling, & M. A. Straus (Eds.), *The dark side of families: Current family violence research* (pp. 69–84). Beverly Hills, CA: Sage Publications.

Warner, J. E., & Hansen, D. J. (1994). The identification and reporting of physical abuse by physicians: A review and implications for research. *Child Abuse and Neglect, 18*, 11–25.

Warren, J. I., Murrie, D. C., Stejskal, W., Colwell, L. H., Morris, J., Chauhan, P., et al. (2006). Opinion formation in evaluating the adjudicative competence and restorability of criminal defendants: A review of 8,000 evaluations. *Behavioral Sciences and the Law, 24*, 113–132.

Warren, J. I., Rosenfeld, B., Fitch, W. L., & Hawk, G. (1997). Forensic mental health clinical evaluations: An analysis of interstate and intersystematic differences. *Law and Human Behavior, 21,* 377–390.

Washington v. Harper, 494 U.S. 210 (1990).

Washington v. United States, 129 U.S. App. D.C. 29 (1967).

Webster, C., Douglas, K., Eaves, D., & Hart, S. (1997). *HCR-20 Assessing risk for violence: version II.* Burnaby, British Columbia: Mental Health, Law & Policy Institute, Simon Frazier University.

Weiler, B. L., & Widom, C. S. (1996). Psychopathy and violent behavior in abused and neglected young adults. *Criminal Behavior and Mental Health, 6,* 253–271.

Weiner, B. A. (1985). The insanity defense: Historical development and present status. *Behavioral Sciences and the Law, 3,* 3–35.

Weiner, I. B., & Hess, A. K. (2006). *The handbook of forensic psychology.* Hoboken, NJ: John Wiley & Sons, Inc.

Werner, E. (2000). Protective factors and individual resilience. In J. P. Shonkoff & S. J. Meisels (Eds.), *Handbook of early childhood intervention* (2nd ed., pp. 115–132). New York: Cambridge University Press.

Wertheimer, A. (1993). A philosophical examination of coercion for mental health issues. *Behavioral Sciences and the Law, 11,* 239–258.

Wetter, M. W., Baer, R. A., Berry, D. T. R., Robison, L. H., & Sumpter, J. (1993). MMPI-2 profiles of motivated fakers given specific symptom information: A comparison to matched patients. *Psychological Assessment, 5,* 317–323.

Wetter, M. W., & Corrigan, S. K. (1995). Providing information to clients about psychological tests: A survey of attorneys' and law students' attitudes. *Professional Psychology: Research and Practice, 26,* 474–477.

Wettstein, R. M., Mulvey, E. P., & Rogers, R. (1991). A prospective comparison of four insanity defense standards. *The American Journal of Psychiatry, 148,* 21–27.

Wexler, D. B., & Winick, B. J. (1991). *Essays in therapeutic jurisprudence.* Durham, NC: Carolina Academic Press.

Wheatman, S. R., & Shaffer, D. R. (2001). On finding for defendants who plead insanity: The crucial impact of dispositional instructions and opportunity to deliberate. *Law and Human Behavior, 25,* 167–183.

Whittemore, K. E., & Kropp, P. R. (2002). Spousal assault risk assessment: A guide for clinicians. *Journal of Forensic Psychology Practice, 2,* 53–64.

Widom, C. S. (1976). Interpersonal and personal construct systems in psychopaths. *Journal of Consulting and Clinical Psychology, 44,* 614–623.

Widom, C. S. (1989). Does violence beget violence? A critical examination of the literature. *Psychological Bulletin, 106,* 3–28.

Wieter v. Settle, 193 F. Supp. 318 (W.D. Mo. 1961).

Weithorn, L. A., & Grisso, T. (1987). Psychological evaluations in divorce custody: Problems, principles, and procedures. In L. A. Weithorn (Ed.), *Psychology and child custody determinations: Knowledge, roles, and expertise* (pp. 157–181). Lincoln: University of Nebraska Press.

Wildman, R. W., Batchelor, E. S., Thompson, L., Nelson, F. R., Moore, J. T., Patterson, M. E., et al. (1978). *The Georgia Court Competency Test: An attempt to develop a rapid, quantitative measure of fitness for trial.* Unpublished manuscript.

Wilkinson, A. P. (1997). Forensic psychiatry: The making-and breaking-of expert opinion testimony. *Journal of Psychiatry and Law, 25,* 51–112.

Subject Index